The 3 Thyroid Plan

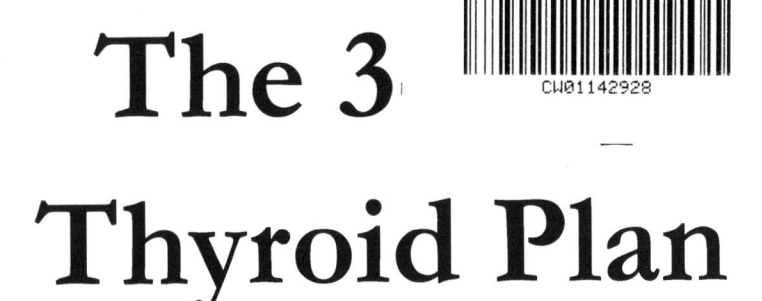

21 Days to Beating Hypothyroidism through Simple Diet and Lifestyle Changes (Now! Includes 40 Delicious Metabolism Boosting Recipes)

Maggie Fitzgerald

LIVENATURAL PRESS

Atlanta, Georgia USA

ISBN 978-1-491010-38-9

All Rights Reserved

No part of this book may be reproduced or transmitted for resale or use by any party other than the individual purchaser who is the sole authorized user of this information. Purchaser is authorized to use any of the information in this publication for his or her own use only. All other reproduction or transmission, or any form or by any means, electronic or mechanical, including photocopying, recording or by any informational storage or retrieval system, is prohibited without express written permission from the author.

Copyright © 2012 Maggie Fitzgerald

Readers' Feedback

"Amazing book! Look no further for the answers you're looking for. The solution is right here!"

★★★★☆ Laura B. - Montreal

"My mother had me read this book after I had a tough time getting rid of my post-pregnancy fat. This book really is an eye opener. I lost all the weight I'd gained, and then some! I've never felt better, and I know my own daughter will grow up a lot healthier and slimmer too!"

★★★★★ Erica Meyer - Washington

"Somehow everything just clicked for me when I read this book. I'm feeling much better, and getting slimmer every day. I can really recommend this book. Buy it and read it if you have any stubborn weight issues."

★★★★★ Joan B. Miller - Sydney

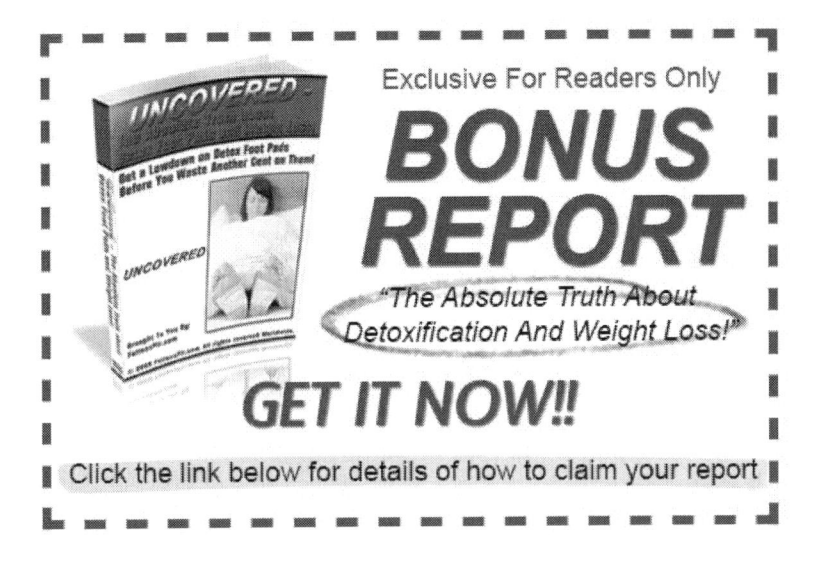

> **Exclusive For Readers Only**
>
> # BONUS REPORT
>
> *"The Absolute Truth About Detoxification And Weight Loss!"*
>
> ## GET IT NOW!!
>
> Click the link below for details of how to claim your report

Exclusive Bonus Download: The Absolute Truth About Detoxification And Weight Loss!

Detoxifying the body is very important for its health and general well-being; yet, the concept is gravely misunderstood by most people. Centuries ago, health masters in the East understood the importance of balancing and detoxifying the body. In contrast, the concept is fairly new to the practitioners of Western medicine!

As the concept of detoxification is becoming popular amount the masses, so are the myths and misinformation concerning its benefits and procedure! Unscrupulous, money-hungry manufacturers of health products aren't making the issue any less confusing for the public.

If you've heard of detoxification and are confused about the conflicting messages out there, this report is the right guide for you!

In this Report, You will discover:

- Why is Detoxification Important?!

- How Detoxification Leads to Weight Loss!

- Do Detox Diets Work?

- Do Detox Foot Pads Work?

- Do You Really Need Detox Diets and Foot Patches?

- Free and Natural Ways to Detoxify Your Body.

And MUCH MUCH MORE!

Download this guide and start shredding fat NOW

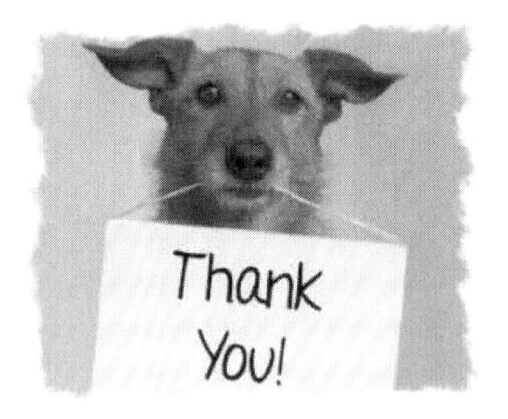

Thank you for downloading my book. Please REVIEW this book on Amazon. I need your feedback to make the next version better. Thank you so much!

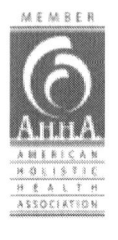

Books by Maggie Fitzgerald

The 14 Day Green Smoothie Detox Diet

The New Green Smoothie Diet

The 3-Step Thyroid Plan

www.amazon.com/author/maggiefitzgerald

Foreword

You should read this book if:

- You feel tired, sluggish and generally run down all the time.
- There's stubborn weight you just can't seem to get rid of - no matter what you do or which diets you try.
- You've been under a lot of stress lately and cannot begin your day without that first cup of coffee.
- You have trouble remembering simple things, like names.
- You've gained weight when normally you have a high metabolism.
- You have cold hands and feet and feel the cold more intensely than others.
- You're tired of being sick and tired.
- You can't seem to think fast and solving simple problems seems difficult.
- You feel depressed without knowing why.
- You've had enough of not feeling your best, and know it's time for a change.
- Feeling comfortable in your own skin is important to you.
- You'd like to enjoy your food without feeling guilty.
- You'd like to join countless others in creating a body which you can show off and be proud off!
- Your romantic life is suffering because you just don't have the energy.

If any of the above rings true, chances are you're suffering from an underactive thyroid. This book will show you exactly what the causes of these symptoms are, and give you a simple and easy step-by-step plan to get you on the road to feeling and looking better than ever.

TABLE OF CONTENTS

Readers' Feedback 2
Foreword 6
Author's introduction 1

CHAPTER 1: HYPOTHYROIDISM AND DIETING 3

1.1. Why Traditional Diets Don't Work 3
1.2. How to Diet Correctly 5

CHAPTER 2: UNDERSTANDING HYPOTHYROIDISM 7

2.1. Thyroid Function 7
2.2. Causes of Hypothyroidism 10
2.3. Symptoms of Hypothyroidism 11
2.4. Diagnosing Hypothyroidism 12
2.5. Treating Hypothyroidism 14
2.6. Hormones 15

CHAPTER 3: THE 3-STEP PLAN 19

3.1. Step 1: Diet 19
3.2. Step 2: Exercise 27
3.3. Step 3: Balancing your Hormones 30
3.4. The 21-day Plan 36

CONCLUSION 43

BREAKFAST 45

1. Turkey Breakfast Sausage 45
2. Blueberry Coconut Pancakes 46
3. Jump Start Granola 47
4. Easy Feta Eggs Scramble 48
5. Choco-Nut Banana Smoothie 49
6. Banana-Almond Porridge 50
7. Gluten-free Breakfast Power Cookies 51
8. Fresh Herbs Omelet 53
9. Carrot 'N Mushroom Frittata 54
10. Crockpot Chicken Meatballs 55
11. Easy Gluten-Free Waffles 57
12. Hazelnut and Almond French Toast 58

LUNCH 61

1. Light Chicken Salad 61
2. Maple Baked Salmon 62
3. Broiled Tilapia over Brown Rice 63
4. Crispy Sole Fish Fillets 64
5. Steamed Cod and Vegetables over Brown Rice 65
6. Creamy Gluten-free Chicken Noodle Soup 67
7. Gluten Free Chicken Piccata Pasta 68
8. Tomato Fish and Veggie Stew 70
9. Cherry Chicken Lettuce Wraps 71
10. Turkey and Jasmine Rice Salad 73
11. Chicken 'N Mushroom Pasta 74
12. Citrus Tuna Steak Sandwich 75

DINNER 79

1. Mozzarella and Spinach Stuffed Cajun Chicken 79
2. Herbed Spaghetti Squash 80
3. Turkey Veggie Stew with Toasted Bread 82
4. Grilled Sea Bass with Lemon Fettuccine 83
5. Gluten-free Chicken and Veggie Stir Fry 84
6. Grilled Spicy Cod with Honey Roasted Carrots 86
7. Pork Chops in Raspberry Sauce with Herbed Basmati Rice 87
8. Teriyaki Salmon with Jasmine Rice 89
9. Gluten-Free Turkey Meat Loaf 90
10. Zesty Olive Chicken with Fried Rice 91
11. Ultimate Spicy Orange Chicken 93
12. Creamy Chicken and Wild Rice Soup 94

DESSERT 97

1. Peach and Triple Berry Parfaits 97
2. Mixed Triple Berry Crisp 98
3. Pumpkin Protein Cookies 99
4. Cranberry Peach Pie 100

EXCLUSIVE BONUS DOWNLOAD: THE ABSOLUTE TRUTH ABOUT DETOXIFICATION AND WEIGHT LOSS! 103

ONE LAST THING 105

Disclaimer

While all attempts have been made to provide effective, verifiable information in this Book, neither the Author nor Publisher assumes any responsibility for errors, inaccuracies, or omissions. Any slights of people or organizations are unintentional.

This Book is not a source of medical information, and it should not be regarded as such. This publication is designed to provide accurate and authoritative information in regard to the subject matter covered. It is sold with the understanding that the publisher is not engaged in rendering a medical service. As with any medical advice, the reader is strongly encouraged to seek professional medical advice before taking action.

Author's introduction

Dieting is hard. I know this from experience—when I was in college, I struggled a bit with my weight. I'd go on one of the fad diets of the day, lose ten pounds, and then gain it back. I'd gain another five pounds. Then I'd lose twenty. Then gain ten back. It was the classic "rollercoaster" pattern of dieting that people talk so much about. I couldn't get my weight under control, and I felt terrible. I was tired all the time, my body didn't feel like it was working properly, and I wasn't sleeping very well. I was really irritable most of the time. This continued after I left college, too. But after six years of this, I decided that enough was enough. I studied to become a nutritionist so that I could determine for myself what was best for me, because the creators of those diets obviously didn't get it. Sure, I could lose ten pounds in a month, but I couldn't keep it off. And I didn't think that losing weight was supposed to make me feel so awful. I knew there had to be something more to it, and after studying and researching, I came to a realization: that traditional diets force us to work against our own bodies, instead of with them. And we were losing the fight.

So I started giving some thought to a better way to diet, and after more studying and research, I settled on one system in the body that was being neglected in every popular diet: the endocrine system, the one that controls our hormones, those chemical messengers that direct most of our body's functions. Not only were we not addressing them, but we were actually hindering their natural functions! Once I figured this out, I knew I had the key to a new way of dieting, one that would address the needs of the *whole* body, instead of just one or two parts. I tried this new method of holistic weight loss, and I was amazed. Not only did it help me lose the weight I had been trying to get rid of for years, and keep it off, but it made me feel so much better than I had felt since long before I had even started dieting! In fact, I'm not sure that I had ever felt as good as I did when I started this diet. Because it's not just dieters that have problems with their hormones—it's everyone. The number of toxins in our food supply is staggering. There are hormone-like substances, inflammatory chemicals, manufactured fats, and a huge number of other things that we just weren't meant to eat. And by removing them from my diet, I started living a new life, one that was happy and healthy.

I knew that I couldn't just keep this secret to myself, but that I had to share it. So here you are—all of my dieting knowledge and experience is condensed into this one book, a simple 21-day plan for cleansing your system of toxins and getting back on track to maintaining a healthy weight. I hope you enjoy this book, that you come to see just how important holistic treatment of excess weight is, and I wish you the greatest success in your weight loss endeavors. Stick with it—you can do it!

Sincerely,

Maggie Fitzgerald

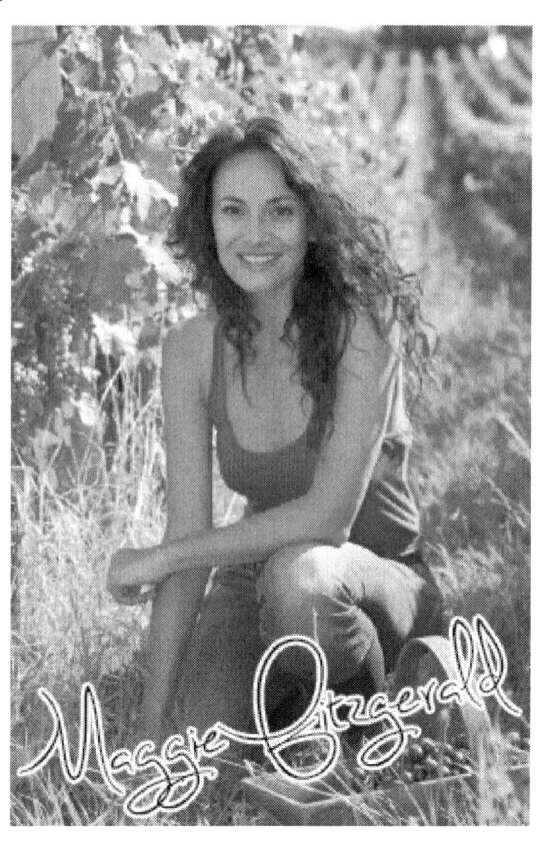

Chapter 1: Hypothyroidism and Dieting

Before going into the details of hypothyroidism and the diet plan, I'd like to take a moment to point out that, in purchasing this book, you're taking a big step toward effective and permanent weight loss. Good work! The relationship between the thyroid and weight loss is so often overlooked, much to our own disadvantage, and by acknowledging the important connection between them, you're starting to view your body as a holistic system, and this is absolutely crucial. So, before we even get started, you're already ahead of the game!

1.1. Why Traditional Diets Don't Work

You probably have experience with ineffective dieting, but do you really understand why it's so hard? Many people think that they just don't have the willpower to stick with a diet, but what they don't realize is that these diets aren't truly effective for several reasons.

First of all, these diets only address your caloric input—this is important, of course, as the only way you're going to lose weight is if you consume fewer calories than you burn. However, that's only a small piece of getting your entire body working for you, instead of against you. This is especially true of the recently popular low-carb diets (like Atkins and South Beach), and is also true of low-protein and low-fat ones as well. If your body doesn't have a proper balanced diet, it won't be able to synthesize the hormones that it needs to function correctly.

The imbalance of nutrients created by these kinds of diets is hugely detrimental to any weight loss efforts. Not only does this kind of dieting actually make it very difficult to lose weight, but it's nearly impossible to keep it off without strictly monitoring many different parts of your life, which takes a lot of time and energy, and doesn't always pay off. If you've done any dieting in the past, you'll know that keeping the weight off and remaining at your ideal weight can be the hardest part, and that you need to very accurately count calories consumed and burned for it to work (if it does at all).

Second, traditional diets don't do anything to address your underlying metabolism. So not only do they cause problems with your hormones, but they also cause your body to burn fewer calories, which means that you'll have to further restrict your caloric intake! It's a really unpleasant cycle that can cause you a lot of stress, which brings me to the third reason that traditional diets don't work—severe calorie restriction can actually cause the release of cortisol, a hormone that can cause a lot of health problems, including increasing the storage of abdominal fat, an unsightly and very unhealthy kind of fat. I'll go into a bit more detail about cortisol in section 2.6. For now, just know that long-term exposure to it is very bad.

Fourth, most traditional diets don't warn you away from "goitrogenic" substances (those that harm the thyroid), but actually recommend consuming *more* of them—things like margarine, diet soda, and sometimes even caffeine. As I'll discuss in section 3.2, these substances should be avoided at all costs, and not encouraged. Many of these foods are linked directly to thyroid dysfunction, which throws your whole body off. Many of these foods are also linked to inflammation, which further increases cortisol release and adverse health effects.

This brings me to the final point, which is that almost all traditional diets recommend drastically reducing your fat intake, which might help you lose weight, but will almost certainly make it more difficult for your body to manufacture the hormones and other chemicals that it needs to work properly. And if you cut out too much fat, you'll also be cutting out fats that are good for you, leading to further inflammation.

As you can see, traditional diets create a self-perpetuating downward spiral that leads to relapsing, difficulty in maintaining your weight, and a number of potentially serious health problems. If you find that diets make you tired, irritable, and maybe even depressed, you're not alone. And it's important to remember that *it's not your fault*. If you haven't had success in weight loss in the past, it's much more likely that you were simply on a diet that was ill-informed and not optimal.

1.2. How to Diet Correctly

Okay, so it's clear that traditional diets aren't going to cut it. Not only do they set you up for failure, but they also may have some serious health consequences. So how *should* you go about dieting? The approach that I'll outline in this book is a holistic one, or one that addresses the body as a complicated system in which each part affects every other part. Holistic medicine has been practiced for centuries, and people are starting to realize that modern healthcare methods might not be the best. My 21-day plan will help you cleanse your body of toxins, start eating a healthy diet, get the exercise you need, and keep your hormones in balance. By combining these elements, you'll help your body to do what it does best—manage itself.

Because of this, you might be surprised at some of the suggestions that are in this book. For example, I don't recommend severely cutting calories, and I don't recommend seriously reducing your fat intake. Instead, I'll encourage you to eat a balanced diet that is nutrient-dense, have your meals at the right time of day, and include a lot of foods that support your immune system. In short, I'm helping you get your diet back to the one that the human body was designed for, instead of the one that's become so popular in the modern Western world--one that's focused on getting as much as we can, as cheaply as we can, and as fast as we can. This is what has led to the obesity and hypothyroid epidemics, and it will continue to damage your health and lead to weight gain unless you do something to stop it.

You may be tempted to combine my recommendations with some of the more traditional styles of dieting—for example, by reducing your intake of carbohydrates. I strongly discourage this, because the guidelines that I've created have been specifically developed to work with each other, and not with other rules. Certain carbohydrates, for example, contain substances that are crucial for reducing the amount of inflammation in your body, and this is a central tenet of this plan. Stick to my guidelines for a month or two, and you'll see why dieting in this way is far superior to the other diets you may have tried in the past.

Chapter 2: Understanding Hypothyroidism

Before getting into the details of my 3-step plan, I'd like to address the issue of hypothyroidism here. Hypothyroidism and other endocrine and metabolic disorders affect millions of people around the world, and may lie at the heart of things like the obesity epidemic and the large number of people who are treated for depression. One 2009 study by Golden et al. stated that 4.6% of Americans over the age of 12 have hypothyroidism. Other figures say somewhere between 10 and 30 million. One of the difficulties with nailing down a specific number is that thyroid disorders often go undiagnosed or are interpreted as a different issue entirely. This makes it especially important that you do whatever you can to prevent, diagnose, and treat this disease. And it's not always a genetic or environmental disorder; Medscape notes that three to five out of every 1,000 women deals with hypothyroidism during pregnancy. Because of these staggering numbers, it's crucial to really understand this disorder.

2.1. Thyroid Function

I'll start with the thyroid gland itself. What is it? First, let's talk about what a gland is. A gland is an organ that secretes a substance—you may have heard of sweat glands, adrenal glands, or sebaceous glands. Well, each of these synthesizes and releases substances into the body, and the thyroid is no different. It's a small gland that's located at the base of your throat, along the midline of your body.

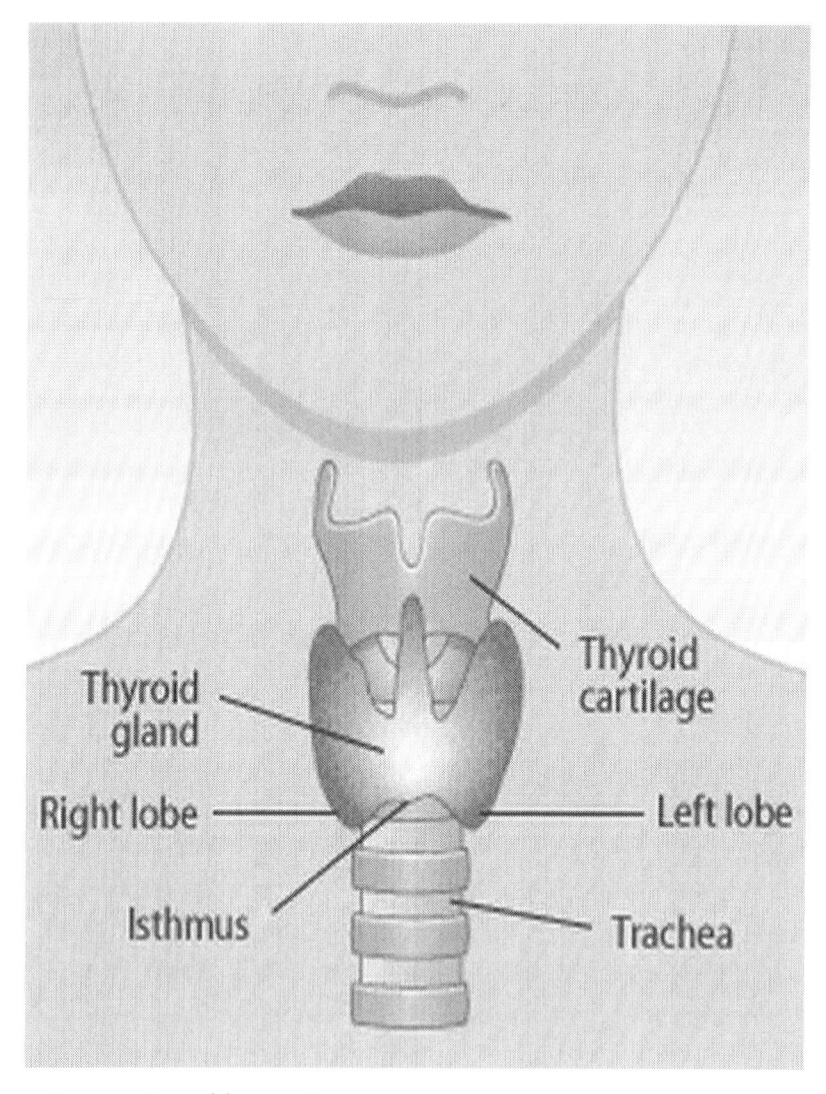

Source: http://www.abc.net.au

Okay, so the thyroid is a gland in the throat. What does it actually *do*? In a nutshell, the thyroid regulates how your body uses energy, which is manifested in your metabolism. You're probably aware of what your metabolism is, but in case you're not, metabolism is the process by which your body turns food into energy. This happens when you eat, but it also happens when you're not eating— and when your metabolism is working correctly, it will use your stored fat for fuel, which leads to weight loss. When your thyroid is working correctly, your metabolism will be going at the proper rate;

conversely, if it's malfunctioning, your metabolism will be improperly regulated, which can lead to your metabolism being too high or too low (hyper- and hypothyroidism, respectively). It's easy to see how this gland makes a big difference in your energy levels and weight loss attempts, and this is why it's so important to make sure that it's functioning correctly. Obviously, this is also very important for overall health; if your body isn't managing its energy correctly, it can have many detrimental effects—some people even think that hypothyroidism is behind many of the common modern, Western diseases, like arthritis and other degenerative diseases, cancer, and some heart disease.

The amount of energy that the cells in your body use is regulated by a hormone called triiodothyronine. When the cells receive it, they'll use more energy. Triiodothyronine is also known as T3, and is produced by the thyroid. The thyroid also produces T4 (thyroxine) that is subsequently converted into T3 by the liver, which actually produces most of the T3 in your body. Moving upwards in the chain, the thyroid is stimulated to produce these hormones by the pituitary gland, which produces TSH, or thyroid stimulating hormone. Prior to this, however, is the hypothalamus, a part of the brain. The hypothalamus monitors a number of things in your body, including the level of thyroid hormones. When more are needed, it produces TSH releasing hormone (TRH) that in turn stimulates the pituitary gland. The pituitary also monitors the level of T3 in the blood, and releases TSH when it becomes too low. Each of these steps is crucial for proper thyroid functioning, and problems with this process can occur at any step (see the next section for more details). Your body also produces reverse T3 (rT3), which is generally produced during times of stress or nutrient deficiency, and can be used as a marker for hypothyroidism.

Once a signal has travelled from the hypothalamus, through the pituitary gland, to the thyroid, more T3 enters the blood stream and kicks your cells into high gear. But sometimes this process goes awry. Hyperthyroidism (overly high amounts of thyroid hormones in the body) is a serious condition, and often shows up with symptoms like heart palpitations, nausea, shakiness, and vomiting. Hypothyroidism, however, is much more common (read on for details on the symptoms of hypothyroidism).

2.2. Causes of Hypothyroidism

When not enough T3 is circulating in your body, you have a condition called hypothyroidism. This can be caused by problems in your hypothalamus, pituitary gland, or the thyroid gland itself. The hypothalamus can become damaged by stroke, a tumor, radiation treatment, and other things that affect the brain. This is much less common, however, than sources of hypothyroidism based in the pituitary or thyroid. If the cause of the problem is in the pituitary, it's likely caused by damage to the gland itself, such as by a tumor or surgery—it's also possible that the pituitary isn't producing enough TSH to stimulate the thyroid. The thyroid itself can also function improperly, and there are a few conditions that might cause this, such as Hashimoto's disease or iodine deficiency.

Hashimoto's disease is an autoimmune disorder that is actually very common—some people even think that most hypothyroidism is caused by this disease. Though the cause is unclear, Hashimoto's causes the thyroid to produce lower amounts of T3 and T4 than it should. Although both hyper- and hypothyroidism can occur without Hashimoto's disease or another autoimmune disorder, scientists are now realizing that most cases include one of these conditions. Another autoimmune disease that affects the thyroid is Grave's disease, but this is much more likely to cause hyperthyroid.

Unfortunately, women are more susceptible to hypothyroidism, as the hormonal changes that we go through throughout our lives (including at puberty, during pregnancy, and after menopause) can throw this system out of whack. Both estrogen and progesterone can affect how the thyroid gland functions, and these are two of the hormones that are in flux during these times. Of course, all of the hormones in the body form a complicated system, and a problem with any one of them can cause issues in the rest (see section 2.6).

There are also some dietary causes of hypothyroidism, including getting too little or too much iodine, which is required for the creation of T3 in the thyroid gland. The recent popularity of low-protein and low-carbohydrate diets also move us away from the balanced diet that is best for our bodies, which causes a number of problems, including hypothyrodism. Fortunately, if you stick with the diet recommendations that I've listed at the end of this book, you should have no problem avoiding dietary causes of hypothyroidism. I've made sure to provide a balanced diet that is high in essential nutrients, contains supplements for other nutrients, and provides the substances your body needs to regulate its hormones.

2.3. Symptoms of Hypothyroidism

As you can see, there are a number of things that can cause hypothyroidism. But what does this mean for those of us who have this condition? Well, there's a very large number of different symptoms that you might be experiencing, and many people have different combinations of these symptoms. Below are some of the most common:

- Lack of energy
- Mental sluggishness
- Mood swings
- Very low metabolism
- Easy weight gain or difficult weight loss
- Cold arms or legs
- Slow recovery from exertion
- Insomnia or poor sleep
- Reduced libido
- Thinning hair on the head or body
- Loss of appetite
- Dry skin and hair
- Hair loss
- Brittle nails
- Acne or rashes
- Dark circles under the eyes

- Swelling in the neck
- Puffiness in the face
- Dry eyes
- Excessive menstrual bleeding or pain
- High cholesterol or blood pressure
- Abnormally fast or slow pulse
- Heart palpitations
- Excessive gas or constipation
- Sweet cravings
- Hypoglycemia

Of course, you may be experiencing symptoms not on this list. If you're just feeling *off*, though, you'll know it, and you might be able to pinpoint a few of these symptoms that could indicate you have a malfunctioning thyroid. And don't ignore what people are telling you—one woman, in discussing her hypothyroidism, said that it was easier for her family and friends to see that something was wrong than it was for her. She also said that mood swings and irritability often just get treated as "that time of the month" for women, who are often considered to be very emotional, and that this can sometimes mask the symptoms. You know if you're feeling right. If not, get yourself checked out!

2.4. Diagnosing Hypothyroidism

If you have a combination of a few of the symptoms listed above, you might be suffering from hypothyroidism, and you should get it checked out. Of course, there are tests that can be done to see if this is the case. If you speak to a doctor about these tests, they're likely to have blood work done. A full thyroid screening will likely test for levels of TSH, free T4, free T3, thyroid antibodies (which may indicate an autoimmune disease) and rT3 (which can signal a disorder called reverse T3 dominance). If you ask a doctor for a thyroid screening and they only test TSH or TSH and T3, you should request a full screening or find a doctor who will give you one, as any single one of these tests may look normal while the rest indicate a disorder. There are also other indicators of hypothyroidism that can be seen by a doctor, such as thyroid nodules, which indicate other types of issues.

In addition to these clinical indicators of the disease, there are a few ways that you can test for hypothyroidism from home. There are a number of labs that now offer hormone testing that only requires you to submit a saliva sample or a very small "blood spot" test through the mail. Saliva tests have been shown to be accurate, and they are significantly cheaper than most blood tests, meaning you should be able to get several different tests done for the price of a single blood test. I recommend having as many hormonal tests done as possible—thyroid hormones, sex hormones, adrenal hormones, and anything else you can get done for a reasonable price. If you're going to be submitting a sample for a test, you might as well get as much as you can out of it! You can find these labs online by running a simple search, or you can try ZRT Laboratory (www.salivatest.com) or Diagnos-Techs (www.diagnostechs.com). Both of these websites have information on the sample submission protocol and testing procedures, and you can always call them to get more information. Also, just for reference, you're probably looking at around $200–$250 for a home test, which might seem like a lot, but is actually quite reasonable compared to what you'd pay at a doctor's office.

An important thing to keep in mind about diagnostics for hypothyroidism is that some people get negative results, and doctors tell them that there's nothing wrong (one woman had an enlarged thyroid, but her doctor couldn't find anything wrong with her thyroid levels, so he told her that she just had a "fat neck"). I can vouch for the fact that this can be really frustrating—but remember that *you* know your body better than anyone else. If you go to a doctor and they tell you that nothing's wrong, you should seriously consider getting a second opinion from another doctor or one of the testing services listed above. Even if hypothyroid isn't at the root of your symptoms, you may find that something else isn't functioning correctly.

2.5. Treating Hypothyroidism

Traditional methods of treating hypothyroidism are like traditional methods of treating everything else—drugs. The most common way to deal with the problem is by prescribing levothyroxine, which is a synthetic version of thyroxine. The thought is that this drug will raise the levels of TSH in your blood, helping your thyroid to get your metabolism back under control. However, there are several problems with this; first and foremost, thyroxine is only one link in the chain of chemicals that manages your metabolism, and the rest of the system must be working correctly to convert it into T3 to stimulate a response. So if your body isn't effectively converting thyroxine into T3 (if your liver isn't functioning properly, for example), more thyroxine isn't going to do you any good. Patients can also experience some really unpleasant symptoms if they take too much levothyroxine. Another prescription for a T3-like drug is available, but it requires multiple doses each day and has a long list of side effects. Other hormone replacement therapies are also used, with varying degrees of success. Bioidentical hormone replacement therapy (BHRT) supplies the body with substances that are chemically identical to the thyroid hormones produced in the body, but this treatment can be hard to find and very expensive.

Medical doctors sometimes get it partly right, though, and recommend additional lifestyle modifications with their prescriptions, including dietary and exercise-related changes. I don't want you to think that every doctor will prescribe ineffective or harmful treatments—it's just that the pharmaceutical industry has a huge amount of money and influence, and this often biases doctors without their even knowing it. This isn't a problem only in hypothyroidism treatments, but in all of medicine. Of course, holistic medicine can't solve *every* problem, but I am a strong believer in the idea that natural and alternative medicines should always be tried before resorting to potentially harmful and disruptive traditional methods. Many people do this the other way around, and start trying natural methods once their pharmaceutical treatments fail, and then discover that holistic therapies are the most effective. You can save yourself a significant amount of time by just skipping the first parts and immediately working with your body using natural methods!

2.6. Hormones

Hormones—we know that they're behind the changes we experience at puberty and menopause, and we blame our teenagers' behavior on them, but what do we *really* know about what hormones do? The endocrine system (which controls hormone production and use) is complicated, and it's involved in a huge number of processes, including metabolism. In this section, I'll give a quick overview of what hormones are and what they do, so that you have a better understanding of why they're so important, both in addressing hypothyroidism and in supporting weight loss.

You've probably heard of a lot of hormones, possibly without even knowing it. Adrenaline, estrogen, progesterone, testosterone, cortisol, serotonin, dopamine, insulin, and melatonin are a few of the hormones that your body creates and uses on a regular basis. Exactly what they're used for differs with each hormone, but to make a sweeping statement, hormones are your body's means of communication. The body is a very complex system, and requires a lot of monitoring and constant adjusting, and the means by which this is done is hormones. When you're facing a stressful situation, you might release adrenaline, making your heart rate rise. When you eat, your brain releases dopamine when you've had enough, signalling that you shouldn't continue eating more. Melatonin helps run your internal clock, making it easier to fall asleep, stay asleep, and get up when you need to. There are a lot of more functions of each of these, and there are many other hormones involved in the endocrine system. As you can see, they're very important.

As I mentioned before, the thyroid hormones affect your metabolism and energy usage. However, it's important to point out that TSH, T3, T4, rT3, and TRH aren't the only things that you need to manage to keep your weight loss efforts on track. For example, if the levels of serotonin in your brain are too low, you might suffer from anxiety, which might cause you to eat more in an effort to relax yourself. You might also feel depressed, which makes many people crave sweets, which can de-rail your weight loss plan really fast. Serotonin also effects digestion. And this is just one hormone! It's obvious why making sure that your entire hormonal system is working correctly is important to managing your hypothyroid. One hormone that I will specifically address here is cortisol. Cortisol is a hormone that is released when you're stressed, either physically or mentally, and helps you cope with that stress *in the short-term*. Long-term exposure to cortisol is related to a huge number of problems, including increased abdominal fat storage, disruption of metabolism, destruction of muscle tissue, reduction of serotonin, and disruption of blood sugar management. Every one of these can not only hugely impact your weight loss efforts, but also have adverse effects on your overall health, including possibly reducing your life expectancy. Cortisol is no joke! Later on, in the 3-step plan that I outline in the second half of this book, I mention stress management as an important step in balancing your hormones, and I hope you understand now why it's such an important step.

Now that you understand why hormones are so important, I'll give a quick overview of which hormones are crucial for healthy weight loss.

1. Thyroid hormones.

I discussed these earlier, but to sum it up succinctly, they manage your body's metabolism.

2. Insulin.

This hormone manages your body's storage and use of fat, making it critically important to losing weight. Having too much insulin in your blood (which can be caused by chronic consumption of sugary, nutrient-poor foods or not having enough fiber or protein in your diet) can result in increased fat storage in the abdomen, more food cravings, and increased storage of water, making you more bloated.

3. Cortisol.

As mentioned a couple paragraphs ago, cortisol is helpful in the short-term, but persistent exposure can result in abdominal fat storage, poor metabolism, and disruption of your blood sugar management, which is controlled primarily by insulin—which means that a problem with cortisol often means a problem with insulin. As you can see, problems with one hormone can throw off the whole system!

4. Estrogen.

Though it's a sex hormone, estrogen has a big effect on your weight loss efforts, as too much estrogen can be a huge risk factor for obesity, and too little can cause more fat storage around your waist. Your mood, memory, and mental acuity are all affected by estrogen, and having an imbalance can put you at greater risk for certain types of cancer. It's important to note that men have estrogen in their bodies as well—it serves crucial functions for everyone.

5. Progesterone.

Another sex hormone, progesterone balances out estrogen in many ways, though too much or too little of it can have a lot of the same effects, including slow metabolism, moodiness, increased stress hormones, autoimmune disorders, and increased risk of certain cancers. Getting estrogen and progesterone balanced is crucial not only for weight loss, but for overall health, both in pre- and post-menopausal women.

6. Neurotransmitters.

I'm simplifying quite a bit by grouping these together, but hormones like serotonin, dopamine, and melatonin (among others) are crucial for sending signals throughout your brain, and play a big role in determining when you're hungry or full, when you're happy or sad, and when you're tired or feeling awake. Chronic stress can really mess with these hormones, so managing your stress will help you get both them and cortisol under control.

7. Testosterone.

Although it's generally considered as a "masculine" hormone, testosterone plays an important role in both men and women—having too little or too much may put you at risk of serious conditions, including heart disease, depression, and osteoporosis. An imbalance in testosterone can also cause unsightly things like acne, facial hair growth, and male-pattern hair loss, even in women.

8. Growth hormone.

This hormone is responsible for repairing and building new cells, and having enough of it can slow the aging process, reduce abdominal fat, help ward off depression, and keep your bones healthy.

Although there are loads more hormones than these eight that affect your body and your weight loss, these are some of the most important, and the ones that will be addressed by the diet recommendations in this book. It's pretty likely—especially if you're having trouble maintaining your ideal weight—that you have an imbalance in several of these hormones. Fortunately, it's pretty easy to fix in a few steps! By performing a cleanse, improving your diet, exercising sufficiently, and taking a few other steps to help balance out your hormones, you'll be well on your way to making your weight loss goal.

Chapter 3: The 3-step Plan

Now that you understood how hypothyroidism and trouble controlling your weight are related, you're ready to start getting into the weight loss plan. By taking a holistic, natural approach to your hypothyroidism for 21 days, you will be well on your way to being healthier, happier, and able to maintain your ideal weight. Of course, the longer you continue the diet and lifestyle recommendations, the healthier you will be, but the initial phase of starting and adjusting to the plan lasts three weeks. After that, all you have to do is keep it up, and you'll keep the weight off! The plan is broken into three parts: diet, exercise, and hormone balance. Each of these, by itself, is critical in your thyroid (and overall) health, but the combination of all three is what's important for really getting your body functioning properly.

3.1. Step 1: Diet

Most of the diet recommendations that I'll give here are ones that you've heard before, especially if you've gone on other diets or if you pay attention to health news. However, this specific combination of dietary guidelines will help you fight the weight gain that can be caused by hypothyroidism. There are many additional benefits to the guidelines, including reduced blood pressure and cholesterol, lower risk of heart disease, decreased chance of stroke and other serious conditions, and reduced chances of developing various degenerative diseases. I can't possibly list all of the benefits of maintaining a healthy, balanced diet based on these guidelines. You'll feel better, you'll look better, and you'll be healthier. You'll just have to see for yourself! (Of course, before starting any diet or taking any supplements, discuss your health with your doctor.)

1. Eliminate harmful foods.

If you're undertaking a diet in an effort to improve your thyroid function, the first thing that you should do is make sure that the foods you're eating don't counteract all of your other efforts. There are many foods that are goitrogenic, or thyroid-damaging, that are often included in other diet plans, and for this reason, I'm setting them out first so you can keep them in mind while you read the other dietary guidelines.

First, avoid gluten. I know this isn't easy—but if you're experiencing weight gain related to hypothyroidism, it will make a huge difference in your weight loss efforts. Not only will it help the hypothyroidism, but eliminating gluten forces you to make healthier choices in general. In case you're not familiar with gluten, it's a substance that's contained in wheat, rye, barley, and some other grains. You'd be surprised at how many other food items contain gluten. Unless the packaging specifically says "gluten-free," don't make any assumptions. Today, many bread products are pitched as being "all natural" or "healthy choices," but some scientists believe that the human body has not evolved enough since the advent of agriculture (sometime around 10,000 or 12,000 years ago) to properly digest gluten. Because of this, it throws the digestive process out of whack and leads to a number of problems, including inflammatory disorders and weight gain. By taking gluten out of your diet, you're taking a major step toward thyroid health and weight loss. At the very least, you should *significantly* reduce your gluten intake.

Second, reduce your intake of both sugar and salt. Very sugary foods make it almost impossible to maintain a steady blood sugar level, meaning you're likely to have severe energy swings. They also cause big shifts in the amount of insulin in your blood. And salty foods can cause problems with fluid retention, which will not only derail your weight loss efforts, but also contribute to higher blood pressure. Once you've eliminated (or significantly decreased) gluten, sugary foods, and salty foods from your diet, you will be left with mostly unprocessed foods that are closer to their natural state, which is easier for your body to digest and extract nutrients from. These are the foods that your diet should consist of—raw, unprocessed, whole foods.

Third, work to ensure that your fat intake is properly balanced. Increase the amount of "good fats" that you consume—these are the fats that are found in things like extra virgin olive oil, oily fish (like salmon and mackerel), and raw seeds and nuts. Polyunsaturated fats, as they are called, contribute to heart health and a reduction of the inflammatory chemicals in your body.

At the same time, you should try to reduce the bad fats in your diet, which are found in things like fatty red meats and dairy products. Choose lean cuts of meat and low-fat dairy to keep the amount of saturated fats down. You should also avoid trans-fats, which have been created by the food industry; they are by far the worst, because they're very unnatural and can't be properly processed by your body. They can also cause serious damage to the membranes of thyroid cells. Trans-fats are found in pre-processed snack foods (like donuts and snack cakes), margarine, and deep-fried foods. Shortening and deep-frying oil are also significant sources of trans-fats. You should aim to have *zero* trans-fats in your diet.

Trans-fats aren't the only food that can be damaging to the thyroid, though. There is actually a certain type of vegetable that can also be problematic. This type, known as "cruciferous" vegetables, causes problems with the creation and function of thyroid hormones and iodine metabolism, both of which are crucial to proper thyroid function and weight loss. Cruciferous vegetables, like cauliflower, cabbage, turnips, Brussels sprouts, and broccoli, should be reduced, but not totally eliminated, as there are many health benefits to be gained from having them in your diet in small quantities. You can also reduce their thyroid-damaging effect by cooking them before you eat them. I know that it seems counterintuitive to avoid vegetables while you're on a diet, and you can get away with not reducing these quite as much as I recommend, but try to only have one serving of cruciferous vegetables per day, and occasional days without any at all, if possible.

In addition to the above guidelines, you should also avoid alcohol, caffeine, and artificial sweeteners. I know that you can't always totally cut these things out of your diet—I definitely understand how much of a life-saver a cup of coffee can be when your kids need to get to practice early in the morning—but reducing them as much as possible will really help you lose weight and keep it off.

2. Control your blood sugar.

In the previous guideline, I mentioned that you should avoid very sugary foods, partly in an effort to control your blood sugar. However, because your blood sugar is one of the strongest determinants of your metabolism and energy levels, it's important to do more than just avoid extra-sugary foods. You should also be conscious with your food choices throughout the day to make sure that your blood sugar stays as level as possible. By doing this, you're making it easier on your hypothalamus, pituitary gland, and thyroid by not asking them to rapidly change your metabolism several times throughout the day. In addition to this, keeping your blood sugar as level as possible is one of the best ways to aid yourself in weight loss, as you'll be less likely to eat unhealthy snacks because you're hungry between meals.

So how do you control your blood sugar? This is one of the most difficult tasks that dieters face. When your blood sugar is low, you get tired and hungry (and, if you're like me, pretty irritable, too). Eating sugary foods causes your blood sugar to spike, making you feel better for a bit, but then they fall back down again, leaving you back where you started. By making good choices in your meals and snacks, you can help your body regulate its blood sugar and energy levels, which helps your thyroid gland do its job. A really helpful concept in managing your blood sugar is the glycemic index, which is a measure of how rapidly a certain food raises your blood sugar. Foods that keep you full and energized longer have lower values on the scale.

Table 2. Glycemic Index for Selected Foods (Relative to Glucose)			
Food	Glycemic Index (Glucose = 100)	Serving Size	Carbohydrate per serving (g)
Dates, dried	103	2 oz (60g)	40
Cornflakes	81	1 cup (30g)	26
Jelly beans	78	1 oz (30 g)	28
Puffed rice cakes	78	3 cakes (25g)	21
Russet potato	76	1 medium (150g)	30
Doughnut	76	1 medium (47g)	23
Soda crackers	74	4 crackers (25g)	17
White bread	73	1 large slice (30g)	14
Table sugar (sucrose)	68	2 tsp (10g)	10
Pancake	67	6" diameter (80g)	58
White rice (boiled)	64	1 cup (150g)	36
Brown rice (boiled)	55	1 cup (150g)	36
Spaghetti, white; boiled 10-15 min	44	1 cup (140g)	33
Spaghetti, white; boiled 5 min	38	1 cup (140g)	40
Spaghetti, whole wheat; boiled	37	1 cup (140g)	37
Rye, pumpernickel bread	41	1 large slice (30g)	12
Oranges, raw	42	1 medium (120g)	11
Pears, raw	38	1 medium (120g)	11
Apples, raw	38	1 medium (120g)	15
All-Bran™ cereal	38	1 cup (30g)	23
Skim milk	32	8 fl oz (250ml)	13
Lentils, dried; boiled	29	1 cup (150g)	18
Kidney beans, dried; boiled	28	1 cup (150g)	25
Pearled barley; boiled	25	1 cup (150g)	42
Cashew nuts	22	1 oz (30g)	9
Peanuts	14	1 oz (30g)	6

Source: prostate-cancer.org

By replacing foods that are higher on the scale with foods that are lower on the scale, you can better control your blood sugar and stay satiated longer. For example, you can replace white bread, which has a glycemix index of 73, with rye bread, which has a significantly lower GI of 41. You'll also note that whole wheat spaghetti is lower than white spaghetti. You can find GI values for a huge number of foods online, and I encourage you to do so. You might be surprised by some of the foods that are really high on the list—rice cakes, for example, are a common traditional diet food, but have a very high value of 78.

As you can see, the foods on the lower end of the scale have some things in common. They're not overly sweet, and they often include two important things: protein and fiber. Having enough protein in your diet is crucial for your thyroid health, as protein is required both for proper liver function and for the stimulating the release of thyroid hormones. Protein also helps you feel full and stay full longer.

The best sources of protein are unprocessed lean meats: things like organic, free-range turkey, for example, or lean cuts of all-natural pork. Eggs are a great source of protein, too, though they have more cholesterol than is ideal. You can also get protein from plant sources, like nuts and soy products, though these aren't quite as beneficial as lean animal sources. If you're a vegetarian, however, you'll have to get more creative with your protein sources and include beans, legumes, and some dairy products to make sure you get the recommended amount of protein every day. The Centers for Disease Control and Prevention recommends 46 grams of protein per day for women, and 56 grams for men.

Fiber serves a similar function in controlling your blood sugar, in that it slows the absorption of calories into your blood stream. By spreading out the absorption of nutrients, fiber helps you stay satiated longer, meaning you won't be going back to the snack cupboard every hour. It also has the added benefit of being very good for your digestive health (in short, it helps clean out your system). All of these things are important in managing hypothyroidism and in weight loss. The Mayo Clinic recommends 30–38 grams of daily fiber intake for men (with younger men towards the higher end of the scale), and 21–25 grams for women (with younger women toward the higher end of the scale).

3. Eat at the right times.

It may surprise you to know that eating at the right times is almost as important as eating the right foods. When you think about it, though, it makes sense: because your thyroid manages your body's response to food intake, it's crucial for your weight loss efforts that you time your meals correctly to optimize that response. If you've tried many different diet plans, you've probably tried quite a few different ways of timing your meals: eating six tiny meals a day, eating two big meals a day, skipping breakfast, having a very large breakfast, having snacks, not having snacks . . . no wonder people get confused about how they should be eating to lose weight! Fortunately, when your thyroid is functioning properly, it will help you eat the right amounts at the right times, so you won't have to worry as much about this as you might think you will.

For example, it's crucial to not skip breakfast. By eating within an hour after you get out of bed, you'll ensure that your thyroid kick-starts your metabolism early in the day, maximizing your calorie burning. By consuming some protein (like eggs or a protein shake) with breakfast, you can also help prevent yourself from getting too hungry throughout the morning, making sure that your blood sugar stays relatively level. Similarly, don't eat in the three-hour window before you go to sleep, as this will throw your body's natural rhythm off. If you're really hungry, you can have a small, healthy snack that's high in protein (I like having a slice of lean deli meat with some low-fat cheese). Another important timing principle is to eat shortly after you complete any sort of workout—this will help your body heal and build muscle that will increase your metabolism.

Also, you should try to eat every three to four hours. This may seem like a lot, but most people can do this with three meals and a light snack or two. This helps keep your blood sugar from dropping too sharply, and will also keep cortisol down, which is extremely important, both for managing your hypothyroidism and for losing weight. If you exercise a lot, you may need to eat more, as your body will be burning more calories; keep this in mind while planning your meals, especially if you participate in intense activities like distance running or rock climbing.

Fortunately, when your hormones are balanced and you're eating well, you won't have to worry too much about correctly timing your meals—your body will just tell you when it needs to eat, and you'll likely be following these guidelines without thinking about it. The cleanse portion of the 21-day plan at the end of this section will help get your hormones back on track, so you should be able to stick to this schedule without much difficulty. If you try this and find it very difficult, you can ease your way into it by making slight adjustments to your current eating schedule instead of just jumping into this one.

4. Create a slight calorie deficit.

Although balancing your hormones will get you a long way toward your goal weight, you may find that you have to do some calorie-counting. Personally, I try to avoid this when at all possible, but sometimes it's just required. If you do find that you need to count calories, I recommend doing it, at most, six days a week, just for the sake of your mental health. Don't overdo it and eat way too much on your days off (you still have to be responsible), but take some time off of obsessively measuring your food.

Of course, the number of calories that you need to eat in a day depends on a lot of things, including your height, weight, and activity level. However, if you're looking for a very rough guide, women probably need around 1500 calories in a day to lose weight, and men need about 2000. I highly recommend using a website like loseit.com (they also have great iOS and Android apps) to get a recommendation on how many calories you should be eating, as well as how many you're burning with your exercise.

You should aim to lose about half a pound each week, which comes out to a 500-calorie deficit each day. This is a reasonable pace to lose weight, and by not undergoing severe calorie restriction, you won't be working against your hormones. This may seem a bit counterintuitive, but if you restrict your calories to a number much lower than your body requires, your metabolism will slow down and you'll produce excess cortisol, which is really counterproductive. This is one of the most serious flaws in traditional diets.

5. Perform occasional cleanses.

In the 21-day plan presented later in the book, I give the details of a two-week cleanse, which will help remove toxins from your body and allow your hormones to get back in balance. Although you might hate doing this for the first few days, it gets better pretty quickly, and you'll quickly start feeling much better. In fact, you might find that you feel better than you ever have before! This is also something that should be done on occasion throughout the time that you spend dieting. I usually do a one-week cleanse once every three months or so. This helps me make sure that my body has flushed out any toxins that I may have inadvertently consumed. Also, if I'm being honest, I sometimes break the rules of my own diet when I'm under a lot of stress—a slice of chocolate cake is great when you're writing late at night and have a deadline the next day! And because of this, I like to continue cleansing on a regular basis. How often you do this is up to you, but I do recommend continuing to do it every once in a while to make sure that harmful substances aren't building up in your body.

3.2. Step 2: Exercise

While dieting is definitely a cornerstone of any weight loss plan, exercise is just as important, especially if you're battling hypothyroidism. When you exercise, your body needs to burn calories to meet your increased energy requirements—this is why it helps you lose weight, but this effect is also beneficial for your thyroid. If your body needs more energy, your metabolism will increase, which requires stimulation from your thyroid; you can think of this as, in effect, exercising your thyroid as well as your muscles. If you have a severe case of hypothyroidism, you might find that exercising is difficult or makes you feel extremely fatigued—if you find that you feel this way, you should talk to your doctor about how to best start an exercise program without exacerbating your current symptoms.

Everyone's exercise needs and preferences are different, so it's a good idea to experiment a bit with your workouts. Below is a list of some of my favourite ways to exercise, and I hope that you'll give at least some of them a try. However, what really matters is that you enjoy what you're doing, because if you like the exercises you do, you'll be a lot more likely to do them. The other advice that I can offer when it comes to exercising is that you should try to find an exercise partner. Whether that's your husband, a friend, your kids, your mom, your cousin, or a co-worker, get someone to set some goals and meet you for exercise on a regular basis. This will keep you accountable and make it more fun to get your calorie-burning exercise in. Many people also find that electronic tracking devices, like the FitBit and the BodyBugg, are very motivating.

1. Walking

Many people are surprised by the fact that walking is often discussed as a really great exercise. But, because it raises your heart rate, uses many different muscles, and requires you to stay upright the whole time, it's actually beneficial in many different ways. Walking increases your metabolism, burns calories, and will help strengthen your bones, which is especially important for women who are approaching menopause, as they may be at increased risk of osteoporosis. One of the reasons why I like walking so much is that you can do it anywhere. Go on a lunch-time walk at work, or walk to the grocery store if you only need milk and eggs, or take the dog on an extra-long walk. Buying a pedometer (or, if you want to spend a little more, a Nike FuelBand) can be a fun way to keep track of how much you walk in a day. Because I've lived in some really outdoorsy places, I've done quite a bit of hiking, and this has become one of my favorite things to do—spending time walking outside in nature is really great for your health, both physical *and* mental. Pack a lunch and make a day of it!

2. Yoga

Though it's generally considered a meditative and reflective activity, yoga can actually be quite taxing, especially if you take a class in a more demanding style, like kundalini or ashtanga yoga. I once attended a yoga for athletes class for a few weeks, and I felt myself getting stronger almost immediately! Not only is it good exercise, but it also targets a lot of the muscles that residents of the modern

Western world neglect, like your abs, back, and hips—the muscles that give you good posture and help you fend off back pain. Yoga is one of my favorite ways to exercise, and it's usually pretty easy to find yoga classes near you, whether at a community center, a university campus, or through a community education program. Also, if you find that you don't like yoga, but you want to do some sort of strengthening, give Pilates a try. Just be ready to be *really* sore after your first few Pilates workouts!

3. Sports

If you're like a lot of the people that I know, when you hear "sports," you think of things like football, basketball, and hockey . . . and immediately think "there's no way I can do that." However, I've introduced quite a few people to tennis and swimming, and a lot of them have really enjoyed both of these activities! I know other people who like to go rollerblading, throw a frisbee, attend aerobics classes, or do some light weight lifting. There are a lot of really fun activities out there that you can try, and I strongly encourage you to try a few of them out. Take a class at a local fitness center, or sign up for a beginner's program through a community education program. It's a great way to meet people, spend some fun time outside, and get your weekly dose of exercise. If you've ever thought that it might be fun to try something new, give it a shot! You have nothing to lose, and you may find a new activity that you really love.

4. Treat other activities as exercise

It's good to remember that not all of your exercise has to come from intense activities. If your car is looking dirty, wash it in your driveway with your kids instead of taking it to the car wash. Park farther away from the store and walk across the parking lot instead of driving in circles looking for a spot close to the store entrance. Take the stairs instead of the elevator. Dance around while you're vacuuming or doing dishes. One of my favorite ways to burn calories without feeling like I'm exercising is to play with my daughters in the park—whether it's running around on the playground, climbing the jungle gym, throwing a ball, or just playing around, it definitely gets my metabolism going. If you think about it, you can make almost everything you do a little more like exercise—before you know it, you'll be burning loads of calories without even thinking about it!

Of course, these are only four ideas for ways to get your heart rate up and your metabolism going. Everyone has their own preferred way, and I encourage you to find what works for you. Whether you start walking, pick up a sport, or take up something totally different, like house painting, you should find something that you really like to do, get out there, and do it!

Now that you have a few ideas on how to add exercise to your schedule, you might be wondering how much exercise you should be doing. The Center for Disease Control and Prevention recommends 2.5 hours of moderate aerobic activity each week (or 1.25 hours of vigorous activity), with two or more days of muscle strengthening activities. However, to make sure that your thyroid is sufficiently stimulated, and to promote consistent weight loss, you should aim for at least 45 minutes, five times a week. Ideally, you should find some way to exercise every day. I know that sounds like a lot, especially if you're working full-time, taking care of your kids, and trying to find time to take care of yourself, but you'll find that it's worth it. I've learned that exercising on a regular basis not only helps me keep weight off, but also makes me feel better—if something comes up at work and I can't exercise for a few days, I start feeling sluggish and unmotivated, and I often get really irritable. Once you get started exercising on a regular basis, it's tough to stop!

3.3. Step 3: Balancing your Hormones

Because your metabolic cycle is driven in large part by hormones, keeping your entire hormonal system balanced is of the utmost importance. Although most weight-loss plans don't address hormones, this is an absolutely crucial step when you're dealing with hypothyroidism, and should not be neglected. You might be able to lose weight without managing your hormones, but if you have hypothyroidism, it'll be very difficult to keep it off. By treating this problem holistically, you'll be much more likely to maintain your weight loss.

The body's hormone system is multilayered and very complex, which means that treating hormonal imbalances often involves doing things that don't seem to be directly related to your thyroid or metabolism—for example, a bit later in this section, I'll discuss why sex is important in starting and maintaining your weight loss. Similarly, estrogen, a hormone that is involved in women's bodily changes in puberty, pregnancy, and menopause, is indicated in many thyroid disorders, and this hormone (along with progesterone) is often taken as an extra supplement by women who are trying to get pregnant. As you can see, the picture starts to get complex very quickly. In this section, I'll give you the basics of getting your hormones back in balance so that your body's natural fat-burning mechanisms can do their job and get you back down to your ideal weight.

1. Get enough micronutrients.

Carbohydrates, proteins, and fats are the main groups of nutrients in your diet (the "macronutrients"). The substances that you need in smaller amounts are called "micronutrients," and include things like vitamins and minerals. If you're eating a healthy, balanced diet, you should be getting all of the micronutrients that your body needs—however, the modern Western diet, which consists mostly of processed foods, is lacking in a lot of the crucial nutrients that your thyroid needs to function properly. Because it's unlikely that you're getting enough of these nutrients, I recommend taking a women's multivitamin.

You can find women's multivitamins at your neighbourhood grocery or department store, but because your body requires high-quality nutrients to combat the effects of hypothyroidism and get your hormones back on track, I strongly recommend visiting a health foods store and buying a high-quality multivitamin like Opti-Women or Now Eve. If you just can't justify spending a bit more money on a high-quality multivitamin, I recommend Women's One-a-Day. There are plenty of options, and the staff at health food stores can help you find what you need. The following vitamins and minerals are especially important:

- Iodine: used by your thyroid to make thyroid hormone.
- Selenium, zinc, copper: used in the T4–T3 conversion process.
- Manganese: involved in T4 production.
- Vitamin A: assists several hormonal processes in the thyroid cycle.
- B vitamins: there are a large number of B vitamins, most of which are involved in regulating your metabolism.
- Vitamin C: used in the synthesis of thyroid hormones.
- Vitamin E: assists in regulating and assisting metabolism.
- Calcium: essential for strong bones, especially for women.
- Folic acid (vitamin B9): crucial, especially before and during pregnancy, for proper fetal development.

Once you have the required micronutrients in your diet, your body will be able to properly synthesize and use hormones, which is the first step in getting them back in balance.

2. Boost fat-burning with anti-inflammatories and anti-oxidants.

Excess inflammation in the body has been linked to all kinds of problems, including the storage of too much fat (and many more sinister things, like degenerative diseases). The Western diet is very high in substances that increase inflammation, but low in anti-inflammatory substances. To combat this, you should include foods in your diet that contain these substances, as well as take supplements to aid your body in reducing inflammation. The most potent anti-inflammatory substance is one that you may have heard of before: omega-3 essential fatty acids.

Omega-3 has become a popular supplement in the recent past as doctors and nutritionists have come to realize its powerful effects on the body. The best sources of omega-3 oils are cold-water fish, like salmon and mackerel, and chia, which is a gluten-free grain that includes a huge amount of this beneficial fat (far more than the fish, in fact). Try to eat this type of fish twice a week, and starting eating chia on a regular basis, and you should be able to get your body's inflammatory response system in check in no time! It's also easy to find eggs that have been supplemented with omega-3, and I recommend these as a great way to get protein into your breakfast as well. If you're looking for supplements that will help you get your inflammation under control, I suggest going with fish oils—if, for some reason, you can't take these, turmeric is also an acceptable anti-inflammatory supplement. Because inflammation is linked to fat storage, if you have it under control, you're much less likely to be storing more fat than you need.

Antioxidants also help alleviate the stress that inflammation causes in the body, and may have other powerful positive effects, such as lowering your risk of developing cancer. Antioxidants are found in many fruits, like tomatoes, watermelon, and pink grapefruit. You can also take antioxidant supplements—again, it's best to go to a health food store and ask the staff there which supplements are best for you. Another source of antioxidants is green tea, so if you're a fan of this wonderful drink, keep it up! Although the caffeine in green tea can be harmful, drinking it in moderation is a great way to get more antioxidants into your diet.

3. Manage stress.

You may not realize it, but stress has a huge effect on your body, not just on your mind. When you get stressed out, your body releases cortisol in response—and while this hormone is helpful in the short term, it can cause a number of detrimental effects if you're exposed to it on a regular basis over a long period of time. Unfortunately, the culture that we've developed places a high value on always being busy and always getting a lot done, which leads to us feeling a lot of pressure and getting stressed when we don't meet the impossible standards that we've set for ourselves. This long-term stress is at the root of a number of health problems, including both heart disease and weight gain—and by managing your stress, you can ensure that hormones of all types, whether it's those that increase fat burning, those that make you feel good, or those that control your appetite, remain in balance.

The first step in managing your stress is to identify your stressors. What stresses you out? Work? Your marriage? Dealing with health issues? Taking care of your parents or your kids? Your health? Taking night classes? Everyone has different stressors, and the best way you can start dealing with them is to make sure that you know which ones are causing you the most difficulty. My favorite way to figure out what's causing stress is to keep a stress journal. Keep a small notebook with you (I find this better than doing it on your phone, as having the actual paper in front of you is more motivating than trying to remember to open up an app) and, whenever you're feeling stressed, jot down a few notes. What are you stressed about? What triggered these feelings? What do you plan on doing about them? And then, later, write down whether or not you were able to successfully deal with this stress and what helped (or hindered) you in this. After a week or two, you should start seeing some patterns emerge, and it'll be easy to identify common stressors.

Once you've identified your stressors, it's time to sit down and make a stress management plan. I know that this doesn't sound like a worthwhile activity, but it can really make a difference. Write down your top three stressors, and jot down two or three ways in which you can manage them. Are you stressed out by the fact that you feel like you're spending more money than you should? Maybe you can make a goal to brew coffee at home three times a week instead of buying a $5 latte. You could also start clipping coupons before you go grocery shopping (or, to save a lot of time, go to coupongeek.com or commonsensewithmoney.com). If you're stressed at your job, you could make a point to be more communicative with your co-workers and your boss about what you can and can't reasonably get done in a 40-hour work week. And so on.

Finally, and maybe most importantly, *make time for yourself*. It may seem a little counterintuitive to take time away from the things you need to get done, but I can speak from personal experience here, and it's crucial to take some time to get away from everything that's stressing you out. Schedule a day at the spa, either for yourself or for you and your girlfriends. Spend a few hours at a local coffee shop with a book and your favorite hot drink. Even just go out walking for an hour. Do *something* to get away from your regular life and reset yourself. This is one of the most important pieces of advice that I can give you. If you're lucky enough to be able to get away for a weekend every now and then, do it!

4. Don't neglect other hormones.

Yes, your thyroid hormones are the ones that are in control of your metabolism, which means that they're extremely important in weight loss. However, you can't just try to fix your thyroid hormones and expect everything to fall into place. If any one of your hormonal systems is out of whack, they're likely all having some problems. Of course, there are many hormonal systems, but there are three that are crucial here: thyroid hormones, sex hormones, and hormones related to exercise. I'll skip the complicated science here, but take my word for it: all three need to be working properly for weight loss, stress relief, and better health. Managing your diet, supplements, and exercise is critical for the thyroid hormones, but this isn't going to do it for the sex hormones! Believe it or not, having good sex on a regular basis (like a couple times a week or more) is important in maintaining your body's hormonal balance. Having sex releases a number of different hormones that have positive effects, like making you feel good, suppressing your appetite, relieving stress, and fighting the effects of aging. Bet you didn't know that sex was *that* good for you! The key thing here is to engage in enjoyable sexual activity—at least two orgasms a week is ideal (note, these don't have to come from a partner!).

Exercising also plays a big role in your hormones, including testosterone, estrogen, and growth hormone, all of which are required for keeping your body in top condition. There are a lot of myths out there regarding exercise among women, so I'll do my best to dispel a few of them here. First, you don't have to worry about "bulking up" from doing exercise (even from lifting weights). Women are naturally smaller than men, and even those who lift weights on a regular basis aren't going to build up tons of muscle. Exercise—including weight lifting—keeps your muscles and bones in good shape. Second, doing hours and hours of low-intensity exercise isn't always the best way to burn calories. Exercise physiologists have found that interval training (alternating short, intense bouts of exercise with longer, more relaxed phases) is actually the most effective for increasing fitness and burning calories. Finally, I'll address one of the myths that is surprisingly common: that very long, very intense sessions of exercise are the most beneficial. If you're pushing your body to the max, you're likely to end up releasing a lot of cortisol and doing a lot of damage. Obviously, this is detrimental to your weight loss and hormonal balance efforts. You shouldn't be totally exhausted at the end of your workouts—ideally, you should be tired, but feel like you could have gone a little while longer.

3.4. The 21-day Plan

Now that you understand the three crucial steps in managing hypothyroidism and meeting your weight loss goals, you're probably getting anxious to start! To help you out, I've provided a plan below that will take you through the three steps in 21 days, starting with a cleanse and ending with a healthy lifestyle that will help get you on track to lose the weight in a healthy, effective, and *permanent* manner. Getting through the first 21 days won't necessarily be easy, but stick with it, and I promise that it'll be worth it! If you can, I definitely recommend doing this with a friend or partner, as it'll be easier than doing it yourself. No matter how you decide to tackle this plan, though, I'm glad that you've made it this far and that you want to get your life and weight under control.

Week 1: The cleanse

Now that you understand how different foods and substances affect your body, I hope you understand why it's so important to cleanse your body of toxins. Your body is generally pretty good at regulating its own hormones, but when we introduce foreign substances into it (especially ones that mimic our own hormones, like estrogen), these processes can get thrown off. Fortunately, you can get this all back under control by going through two weeks of a cleansing diet. This will help you get back on track and lay the foundation for your weight loss. Unlike some cleanse diets, this one consists mostly of eliminating foods that might be contributing to an imbalance in your hormones, and especially your thyroid hormones.

The following list includes all of the foods that you should avoid:

- Gluten-containing grains (wheat, barley, rye), and anything that might include them; if you're going to be consuming grains, make absolutely sure that they are completely gluten-free. You can replace gluten-containing grains with other grains and pseudograins, like quinoa, rice, buckwheat, and amaranth, though you should keep your consumption of these to a moderate level. Most of your carbohydrates should come from produce.
- Red meat should be totally removed from your diet, and replaced with poultry and fish.
- Dairy products should also be mostly removed. You can have a bit of sheep or goat milk or yogurt, though minimize this as much as possible. You can also have plant-derived milks, like soy, almond, and hazelnut milk.
- Vegetable oil and other hydrogenated oils—replace all of your cooking oils with extra-virgin olive oil, avocado oil, or canola oil.
- Added sugar and artificial sweeteners; you won't be able to totally cut sugar out of your diet, but minimize it as much as possible by not eating sugary foods or adding table sugar to anything. If you desperately need some sweetener, you can have a *tiny* amount of stevia.
- Caffeine and alcohol are totally out—no coffee or tea, no beer or wine. These have to go. You can have moderate amounts later, but none during the cleanse.

I know that this includes a lot of foods that are really common in your diet, but once you've gone through two weeks of this, you may be tempted to not start eating them again! Many people find that once they start this cleanse, the pounds start coming off, and they feel a lot better than they did before. A couple things that you can do to help ensure that you're not going to be really hungry all the time is to drink a lot of water (and I mean *a lot*—try to be sipping on a glass or a bottle of water pretty much all day) and to make sure you're getting a lot of fiber (which also helps the detoxifying process). You should also start taking an omega-3 supplement, like fish oil, and a probiotic supplement probably isn't a bad idea, either.

The best way to start the cleanse is right before you go on a big grocery shopping trip—you should be mostly out of the foods that you need to eliminate, and you can commit to not buying them while you're shopping. That way, you won't have them at home, meaning you'll have less temptation to deal with throughout the two weeks. Finally, I'll note that you may experience lightheadedness or headaches, nausea, gastrointestinal discomfort, or some other minor symptoms during the cleanse. This is just your body getting rid of the toxins. They'll resolve soon, and you'll be feeling better than ever.

Week 2: Adding exercise

Once you've gone through seven days of the cleanse, you should start feeling a lot better. If you're like most people, you'll find that you have more energy, you're happier, and you just generally feel *better*. You may also be finding that sticking to the cleanse diet isn't easy— you have to cut out a lot of foods that are really common in most people's diets. But hang in there! You only have to be on the full cleanse diet for two weeks, and then you get to start adding foods back in. This week, however, you're going to concentrate on staying on the cleanse, as well as adding some exercise to your daily routine. The exact amount is up to you, and depends on how much time you're able to commit and what you like to do, but I strongly recommend that you exercise at least 30 minutes five times this week. If you haven't been exercising at all, start with three times a week, and work up from there. Here are a few tips to help you out.

- Add exercise to your schedule. A lot of people use Google Calendar or iCal to plan out their weeks, and if you do, you should put exercise on it. It'll make you more likely to actually

- get out there and do it when the time comes (plus, you won't forget about it).
- Try something new this week—challenge yourself. If you usually walk for your exercise, try going on a bike ride. If you've been wanting to play badminton again for years, join a local group or challenge your spouse to a game at the local park. Play a new outdoor game with your kids.
- Make a point to integrate some exercise into your life every day—whether that's going for a 15-minute walk to take a quick break from work, taking the stairs instead of the elevator, carrying some heavy pots around your garden, or moving around more while you're cleaning, keep your thyroid healthy by revving up your metabolism.
- Finally, have fun! If you're treating exercise like a chore, you're probably not doing something that you really enjoy. So find something that you love to do, because it will make your dieting more fun and more effective.

Obviously, you won't go from totally inactive to a fitness superstar overnight. But getting started early in your dieting is really important, especially when it comes to your thyroid. Combining the cleanse and the exercise will really help rid your system of toxins, too, setting the stage for the final week of the plan and the rest of your dieting. Continue your water intake and omega-3 supplementation, and your probiotic if you started one, too.

Week 3: The long-term diet

Congratulations! You've made it through the cleanse. Starting in week three, you can begin adding foods, one at a time, back into your diet. Once you add a food, wait a few days until you add another one to see if you have any adverse effects. This is a great way to see if you're sensitive to anything (this is also how many people find that they have minor allergies that they never knew about). For example, on the first day of week 3, you can add a bit of yogurt back into your diet. If you're feeling alright with that, you can add some cheese a couple days later. A few days after that, have a bit of red meat. And so on. In addition to this, it's time to start focusing on the guidelines from the previous sections. Make sure you're getting enough of the anti-inflammatories and anti-oxidants that I listed, and start taking a high-quality multivitamin to ensure that you're getting your micronutrients. Establish a small, but consistent, calorie deficit every day. By putting these things together, you should have no problem getting your hormones balanced out and well on your way to your weight loss goal.

Although they don't cover all of the guidelines that I outlined in the previous section, I have put together this list of the five most important things you can do during this phase of your diet.

1. Eat a lot of fruits and vegetables—five servings a day, if not more. In addition to helping you get your vitamins, minerals, and anti-inflammatory substances, they'll also help keep you full without pushing your calorie count up too high. Have at least one serving with every meal, and snack on some vegetables in the afternoon when you need it. (Remember to keep cruciferous vegetables to a minimum, though).
2. Get enough protein and fiber. Many dieters think that meat is loaded with calories and fat, and try to avoid it as much as possible. But by adding lean meats (like poultry and fish) to your diet, you'll stay satiated longer, and the protein that you get from them will help in the creation of the all-important hormones in your body. Fiber, in addition to helping you stay full, is crucial for your digestive health.
3. Continue with the gluten-free diet. I know it's not easy at first, but gluten can wreak havoc with your body, especially if you have an intolerance that you're not aware of.
4. Try to eat as many organic foods as possible. They're more expensive, but they're also free of pesticides, hormones, and antibiotics, all of which can be damaging both to your body and your weight loss efforts. If you enjoy gardening, try growing a bit of your own food!
5. Don't let yourself get too hungry at any point of the day. Have three or four smaller meals and a snack to help keep your blood sugar level.

If you can stick to these five rules, your hormones will be better managed, and you'll be on your way to permanent weight loss. One of the best ways that you can follow these rules is to use the recipes that I've provided in the back of this book, each of which I have personally looked over to make sure that they meet these guidelines. Of course, there are tons of cookbooks that you can find out there, including organic ones, gluten-free ones, and healthy dieting ones, that will help you on your weight loss path.

Conclusion

Good work! You've made it all the way through the main portion of the book. You understand what the thyroid does, what causes it to malfunction, what that malfunction does, how to get thyroid problems diagnosed, and how to treat hypothyroidism the natural way. You've read the guidelines for a successful diet that will help you get your hypothyroidism under control, as well as help you lose weight and keep it off. You have some ideas on how to get more exercise into your life. And, maybe most importantly, you have a really good understanding of how to keep your hormones, those all-important chemical messengers in your body, in proper balance.

By using all of this knowledge, I am confident that you'll be able to meet your weight loss goals and feel great! There might be some days when you feel like it's not working, and some days when it just seems like too much work, but stick with it, and you'll get through the tough days (trust me, I know how difficult they are!).

In the following sections, I've provided a number of different recipes that you can use for the diet and hormonal balance portions of my 3-step plan. The recipes listed here have the right number of calories, and the proper balance of nutrients, to keep you full and energized, as well as provide your endocrine system with the building blocks that it needs to create and manage hormones. Of course, there are tons of resources online where you can find additional recipes, too. I encourage you to experiment and find what you like!

Finally, remember that you're not the only one dealing with these issues. There are millions of people who deal with hypothyroidism every day, and many of them don't know how to deal with it. Share your knowledge, and improve the lives of other people with hypothyroidism—we can beat it if we work together!

BREAKFAST

1. Turkey Breakfast Sausage

Servings: 8
Preparation time: 15 minutes
Cook time: 10 minutes
Ready in: 25 minutes

Nutrition Facts

Serving Size 59 g

Amount Per Serving	
Calories 135	Calories from Fat 68
	% Daily Value*
Total Fat 7.5g	12%
Saturated Fat 1.9g	10%
Trans Fat 0.0g	
Cholesterol 58mg	19%
Sodium 642mg	27%
Total Carbohydrates 0.6g	0%
Protein 15.6g	
Vitamin A 1% • Vitamin C 0%	
Calcium 2% • Iron 7%	

Nutrition Grade B
* Based on a 2000 calorie diet

Ingredients
- 1 teaspoons ground sage
- 1 tablespoon Stevia
- 2 teaspoons iodized salt
- 1 teaspoon ground black pepper
- 1/4 teaspoon garlic powder
- 1/4 teaspoon dried marjoram
- 1/2 teaspoon crushed red pepper flakes
- 1/8 teaspoon nutmeg
- 1 1/2 teaspoon fennel seed

- 1 pound ground turkey
- 1 tablespoon extra-virgin olive oil, for greasing

Directions
1. **Combine** all ingredients, except the olive oil, in a large bowl.
2. **Shape** mixture into patties.
3. **Grease** a large skillet with the olive oil and place over medium high heat.
4. **Sauté** the patties in the skillet for 5 minutes each side, until they are no longer pink inside and internal temperature reaches 160 degrees F.

2. Blueberry Coconut Pancakes

Servings: 5
Preparation time: 10 minutes
Cook time: 20 minutes
Ready in: 30 minutes

Nutrition Facts
Serving Size 165 g

Amount Per Serving
Calories 350 — Calories from Fat 171

	% Daily Value*
Total Fat 19.0g	29%
Saturated Fat 14.0g	70%
Trans Fat 0.0g	
Cholesterol 131mg	44%
Sodium 523mg	22%
Total Carbohydrates 38.4g	13%
Dietary Fiber 5.8g	23%
Sugars 28.0g	
Protein 7.3g	

Vitamin A 4% • Vitamin C 7%
Calcium 5% • Iron 11%

Nutrition Grade D+
* Based on a 2000 calorie diet

Ingredients
- 4 (omega-3)eggs, room temperature
- 1 cup coconut milk
- 1 tablespoon raw honey
- 2 teaspoons pure vanilla extract
- 1/2 cup coconut flour

- 1 teaspoon baking soda
- 1/2 teaspoon iodized salt
- 1/4 teaspoon ground cinnamon
- 1 cup blueberries
- 1 tablespoon coconut oil, for greasing
- 1/2 cup maple syrup

Directions
1. **Beat** together the eggs in a large bowl until frothy; then add the milk, honey, and vanilla.
2. **Whisk** together coconut flour, baking soda, iodized salt and cinnamon. Add the flour mixture to the egg mixture and beat to combine.
3. **Stir** in the blueberries and let the batter sit for about 2 minutes.
4. **Grease** a pan with coconut oil and put pan over medium-low heat. Pour batter onto pan, about 3 tablespoons for each pancake. Cook for 2-3 minutes on both sides.
5. **Serve** hot and top each pancake with 1 tablespoon maple syrup.

3. Jump Start Granola

Servings: 10
Preparation time: 15 minutes
Cook time: 20 minutes
Ready in: 35 minutes

Nutrition Facts

Serving Size 110 g

Amount Per Serving

Calories 388	Calories from Fat 203
	% Daily Value*
Total Fat 22.5g	35%
Saturated Fat 1.9g	10%
Trans Fat 0.0g	
Cholesterol 0mg	0%
Sodium 2mg	0%
Total Carbohydrates 41.7g	14%
Dietary Fiber 6.6g	26%
Sugars 18.4g	
Protein 8.7g	
Vitamin A 12%	Vitamin C 6%
Calcium 6%	Iron 15%

Nutrition Grade C

* Based on a 2000 calorie diet

Ingredients
- 3 cups gluten free rolled oats
- 2 cups dried apricots
- 1 cup almonds, sliced
- 1 cup pecans, chopped
- 1 cup raw sunflower seeds
- 1/2 cup raw honey
- 1/4 cup canola oil
- 1 tablespoon ground cinnamon
- 1 teaspoon pure vanilla extract

Directions
1. **Preheat** oven to 300 degrees F (150 degrees C).
2. **Combine** oats, apricots, almonds, pecans, and sunflower seeds in a bowl.
3. **Stir** together the honey, canola oil, cinnamon, vanilla in a separate bowl and pour into oats mixture.
4. **Spread** mixture onto baking sheet.
5. **Bake** for 20 minutes, stir halfway through.
6. **Allow** granola to cool completely then serve.

4. Easy Feta Eggs Scramble

Servings: 2
Preparation time: 10 minutes

Cook time: 8 minutes
Ready in: 18 minutes

Nutrition Facts

Serving Size 233 g

Amount Per Serving

Calories 251	Calories from Fat 153
	% Daily Value*
Total Fat 17.0g	26%
Saturated Fat 4.4g	22%
Trans Fat 0.0g	
Cholesterol 358mg	119%
Sodium 376mg	16%
Total Carbohydrates 5.9g	2%
Dietary Fiber 3.1g	12%
Sugars 1.5g	
Protein 16.3g	
Vitamin A 13%	Vitamin C 11%
Calcium 9%	Iron 10%

Nutrition Grade B-

* Based on a 2000 calorie diet

Ingredients

- 1 tablespoon extra-virgin olive oil
- 2 cloves garlic, crushed and chopped
- 1/4 cup onion, chopped
- 4 (omega-3) eggs, beaten
- 1/4 cup tomatoes, chopped
- 2 tablespoons crumbled feta cheese
- 1 dash iodized salt
- 1 dash pepper
- 1 handful spinach leaves

Directions
1. **Heat** olive oil in a skillet over medium heat.
2. **Sauté** garlic and onions until garlic is lightly brown.
3. **Add** the beaten eggs and cook for 1 minute.
4. **Stir** in tomatoes, feta cheese, spinach, salt, and pepper; cook until egg is set and spinach is wilted.

5. Choco-Nut Banana Smoothie

Servings: 4
Preparation time: 8 minutes

Nutrition Facts

Serving Size 240 g

Amount Per Serving

Calories 395	Calories from Fat 161

% Daily Value*

Total Fat 17.9g	**28%**
Saturated Fat 4.3g	**21%**
Trans Fat 0.0g	
Cholesterol 5mg	**2%**
Sodium 213mg	**9%**
Total Carbohydrates 51.7g	**17%**
Dietary Fiber 5.0g	**20%**
Sugars 32.3g	
Protein 13.4g	

Vitamin A 7%	Vitamin C 17%
Calcium 17%	Iron 5%

Nutrition Grade B-

* Based on a 2000 calorie diet

Ingredients
- 4 banana, sliced
- 2 cups low-fat goat's milk
- 1/2 cup peanut butter
- 1 teaspoon raw honey
- 1 cup crushed ice

Directions

Place ingredients in a blender and blend until smooth. Pour into glasses and serve.

6. Banana-Almond Porridge

Servings: 4
Serving size: 1 medium bowl
Preparation time: 8 minutes
Cook time: 4 minutes
Ready in: 12 minutes

Nutrition Facts

Serving Size 185 g

Amount Per Serving

Calories 396	Calories from Fat 169
	% Daily Value*
Total Fat 18.7g	**29%**
Saturated Fat 1.2g	**6%**
Trans Fat 0.0g	
Cholesterol 0mg	**0%**
Sodium 75mg	**3%**
Total Carbohydrates 55.4g	**18%**
Dietary Fiber 8.1g	**33%**
Sugars 35.3g	
Protein 9.5g	
Vitamin A 6% •	Vitamin C 9%
Calcium 12% •	Iron 13%

Nutrition Grade A-

* Based on a 2000 calorie diet

Ingredients
- 2 cups low-fat almond milk
- 2 bananas, mashed
- 3/4 cup almond meal
- 1/4 cup flax meal
- 1/2 cup raw almonds, sliced
- 1 teaspoon raw honey
- 1 teaspoon ground cinnamon
- 1/4 cup organic pure maple syrup
- 1/2 cup raisins

Directions
1. **Heat** milk in a saucepan over medium heat.
2. **Stir** in almond meal, flax meal, almonds, bananas, and honey until smooth. Sprinkle cinnamon over mixture.
3. **Simmer** for about 3-4 minutes, or until thick and bubbly.
4. **Ladle** porridge into bowls. Add raisins on top then drizzle with maple syrup.

7. Gluten-free Breakfast Power Cookies

Servings: 6
Preparation time: 25 minutes
Cook time: 15 minutes
Ready in: 40 minutes

Nutrition Facts

Serving Size 144 g

Amount Per Serving

Calories 414	Calories from Fat 205
	% Daily Value*
Total Fat 22.8g	**35%**
Saturated Fat 7.8g	**39%**
Trans Fat 0.0g	
Cholesterol 0mg	**0%**
Sodium 188mg	**8%**
Total Carbohydrates 46.3g	**15%**
Dietary Fiber 6.3g	**25%**
Sugars 20.8g	
Protein 11.6g	
Vitamin A 1% • Vitamin C 6%	
Calcium 6% • Iron 14%	

Nutrition Grade F

* Based on a 2000 calorie diet

Ingredients
- 2 medium ripe bananas, mashed
- 2 tablespoons ground flaxseed
- 5 tablespoons water
- 1/2 cup low-fat salted peanut butter
- 2 tablespoons applesauce
- 3 tablespoons raw honey
- 1 teaspoon pure vanilla extract
- 1 pinch iodized salt
- 1 1/2 cup gluten free rolled oats
- 1 cup almond flour
- 1/2 teaspoon baking powder
- 1/2 teaspoon baking soda
- 1/2 cup dark chocolate chips
- Coconut oil for greasing

Directions
1. **Preheat** oven to 350 degrees F. Lightly grease a baking sheet with coconut oil.
2. **Combine** the oats and almond flour in a large bowl.
3. **Mix** ground flax seed and water in a small bowl, let rest for 5 minutes, and then add to the oat mixture.
4. **Add** the mashed banana, peanut butter, baking powder, baking soda, applesauce, honey, vanilla, and salt.

5. **Stir** in chocolate chips. Refrigerate batter for 5 minutes. Scoop and drop batter 2-inches apart onto the prepared baking sheet, using a cookie scoop.
6. **Bake** cookies for 15-17 minutes, or until slightly golden brown.
7. **Remove** from oven and let cool in a wire rack.
8. **Store** cookies in a tightly covered cookie jar.

8. Fresh Herbs Omelet

Servings: 3
Preparation time: 8 minutes
Cook time: 5 minutes
Ready in: 13 minutes

Nutrition Facts

Serving Size 397 g

Amount Per Serving

Calories 211	Calories from Fat 129

	% Daily Value*
Total Fat 14.4g	**22%**
Saturated Fat 4.0g	**20%**
Trans Fat 0.0g	
Cholesterol 6mg	**2%**
Sodium 645mg	**27%**
Total Carbohydrates 9.9g	**3%**
Dietary Fiber 2.9g	**12%**
Sugars 5.6g	
Protein 13.2g	

Vitamin A 6%	•	Vitamin C 79%
Calcium 10%	•	Iron 22%

Nutrition Grade B-
* Based on a 2000 calorie diet

Ingredients
- 1 tablespoon extra-virgin olive oil
- 4 (omega-3)eggs, lightly beaten
- 5 cherry tomatoes, halved
- 2 tablespoons red onions, chopped
- 1 tablespoon fresh dill, snipped
- 1 tablespoon fresh chives, chopped
- 1 tablespoon fresh parsley, chopped
- 1 teaspoon jalapeno, chopped
- 1/4 cup low-fat parmesan cheese, shredded
- 1/2 teaspoon iodized salt, or to taste

- 1/2 teaspoon pepper, or to taste

Directions
1. **Beat** eggs in a large bowl. Add the remaining ingredients, except the olive oil.
2. **Heat** olive oil in a nonstick skillet.
3. **Pour** egg mixture into the skillet and cook for about 2-3 minutes, or until set underneath.
4. **Heat** the broiler.
5. **Place** skillet under the broiler and cook omelet for 2 minutes, or until golden on top.
6. **Slice** omelet into wedges, transfer to a plate and serve.

9. Carrot 'N Mushroom Frittata

Servings: 3
Preparation time: 10 minutes
Cook time: 25 minutes
Ready in: 35 minutes

Nutrition Facts

Serving Size 250 g

Amount Per Serving	
Calories 247	Calories from Fat 138
	% Daily Value*
Total Fat 15.4g	24%
Saturated Fat 3.0g	15%
Trans Fat 0.0g	
Cholesterol 350mg	117%
Sodium 422mg	18%
Total Carbohydrates 10.1g	3%
Dietary Fiber 3.0g	12%
Sugars 4.8g	
Protein 14.1g	
Vitamin A 148%	Vitamin C 66%
Calcium 8%	Iron 23%
Nutrition Grade A-	
* Based on a 2000 calorie diet	

Ingredients
- 1 1/2 tablespoon extra-virgin olive oil
- 1 cup mushrooms, diced
- 1 cup carrots, chopped
- 1/2 red bell pepper, diced
- 1/2 red onion, chopped

- 1 tablespoon fresh thyme, chopped
- 1/2 teaspoon iodized salt, or to taste
- 1/4 teaspoon freshly ground black pepper, or to taste
- 2 cloves garlic, chopped
- 1 medium tomato, seeded and chopped
- 6 (omega-3)eggs

Directions
1. **Heat** olive oil in a medium oven-proof skillet over medium heat. Add garlic and sauté until lightly browned.
2. **Add** mushrooms, carrots, thyme, onion, red bell pepper, and 1/8 teaspoon salt. Cover and cook for about 6 minutes, or until tender. Add tomato and cook for additional 5 minutes.
3. **Beat** together eggs, 1/8 teaspoon salt, and pepper in a medium bowl until frothy.
4. **Gently** pour egg mixture over vegetable mixture in the skillet. Reduce heat to medium-low. Cover and cook for 15 minutes.
5. **Preheat** broiler to low. Cook frittata for 3 minutes under the broiler, or until set.
6. **Transfer** the frittata to a plate, slice, and serve.

10. Crockpot Chicken Meatballs

Servings: 7
Preparation time: 20 minutes
Cook time: 7 hours on LOW
Ready in: 7 hours 20 minutes

Nutrition Facts

Serving Size 245 g

Amount Per Serving

Calories 275	Calories from Fat 119
	% Daily Value*
Total Fat 13.2g	**20%**
Saturated Fat 4.2g	**21%**
Trans Fat 0.0g	
Cholesterol 118mg	**39%**
Sodium 176mg	**7%**
Total Carbohydrates 16.8g	**6%**
Dietary Fiber 4.3g	**17%**
Sugars 8.8g	
Protein 23.3g	
Vitamin A 156% •	Vitamin C 42%
Calcium 8% •	Iron 26%

Nutrition Grade B

* Based on a 2000 calorie diet

Ingredients
- 2 pounds free-range ground chicken meat
- 1 1/2 cup carrots, chopped
- 1 large onion, chopped
- 3 (omega-3)eggs
- 1/2 cup almond meal
- 1 teaspoon dried thyme
- 3 cloves garlic, minced
- 1/8 teaspoon ground black pepper
- 1 teaspoon raw honey
- 2 cups tomatoes, crushed
- 1 cup organic tomato paste
- 1/2 cup fresh parsley leaves, chopped
- 5 cloves garlic, coarsely chopped
- 1/8 teaspoon iodized salt
- 1 pinch of black pepper

Directions
1. **Combine** first 9 ingredients in a large bowl. Shape mixture into large meatballs and place into the crockpot.
2. **Mix** the crushed tomatoes, tomato paste, parsley, garlic, salt, and pepper in a medium bowl.
3. **Pour** the tomato mixture over the meatballs. Cook on Low for 7 hours.

11. Easy Gluten-Free Waffles

Servings: 3
Preparation time: 10 minutes
Cook time: 15 minutes
Ready in: 25 minutes

Nutrition Facts
Serving Size 278 g

Amount Per Serving
Calories 368 — Calories from Fat 182

	% Daily Value*
Total Fat 20.2g	31%
Saturated Fat 11.3g	57%
Trans Fat 0.0g	
Cholesterol 164mg	55%
Sodium 264mg	11%
Total Carbohydrates 41.9g	14%
Dietary Fiber 7.7g	31%
Sugars 22.6g	
Protein 10.2g	

Vitamin A 6% • Vitamin C 26%
Calcium 7% • Iron 13%

Nutrition Grade C
* Based on a 2000 calorie diet

Ingredients
- 3 (omega-3) eggs, room temperature
- 1 cup almond flour
- 1/4 cup coconut milk
- ¼ teaspoon iodized salt
- 1 teaspoon pure vanilla extract
- 1 teaspoon pure maple syrup
- 1 teaspoon cinnamon
- 2 tablespoons coconut butter
- coconut oil, for greasing
- 3 ripe bananas, sliced
- 1 cup frozen blueberries

Directions
1. **Grease** waffle iron with coconut oil and preheat.
2. **Whisk** together the eggs, almond flour, coconut milk, salt, vanilla, maple syrup, cinnamon, and coconut butter until smooth.

3. **Scoop** enough batter onto the waffle iron. Close the lid and cook waffle until golden brown.
4. **Serve** topped with banana slices and blueberries.

12. Hazelnut and Almond French Toast

Servings: 6
Serving size: 2 slices
Preparation time: 15 minutes
Cook time: 30 minutes
Ready in: 45 minutes

Nutrition Facts

Serving Size 119 g

Amount Per Serving	
Calories 305	Calories from Fat 142
	% Daily Value*
Total Fat 15.8g	24%
Saturated Fat 1.8g	9%
Trans Fat 0.0g	
Cholesterol 82mg	27%
Sodium 59mg	2%
Total Carbohydrates 33.4g	11%
Dietary Fiber 4.8g	19%
Sugars 4.5g	
Protein 5.8g	
Vitamin A 2%	Vitamin C 1%
Calcium 134%	Iron 62%
Nutrition Grade C	
* Based on a 2000 calorie diet	

Ingredients
- 3 (omega-3)eggs
- 1/4 cup almond flour
- 1 cup hazelnut milk
- 1 pinch iodized salt
- 1/2 teaspoon ground cinnamon
- 1 teaspoon pure vanilla extract
- 1 tablespoon raw honey
- Coconut oil, for greasing
- 12 thick slices gluten-free bread
- 1/2 cup hazelnuts, finely chopped
- 1/2 cup almonds, finely chopped

Directions
1. **Whisk** together the eggs, almond flour, milk, salt, cinnamon, vanilla, and honey in a large bowl, until smooth.
2. **Combine** chopped almonds and hazelnut in a separate bowl.
3. **Grease** a griddle with coconut oil and put over medium heat.
4. **Soak** bread slices in egg mixture, and then dip one side in the nut mixture.
5. **Place** bread slices in the griddle, nut side down and cook for 5 minutes on each side, or until golden brown. Serve warm.

LUNCH

1. Light Chicken Salad

Servings: 10
Preparation time: 20 minutes

Nutrition Facts

Serving Size 129 g

Amount Per Serving	
Calories 318	Calories from Fat 193
	% Daily Value*
Total Fat 21.4g	33%
Saturated Fat 3.1g	16%
Trans Fat 0.0g	
Cholesterol 48mg	16%
Sodium 537mg	22%
Total Carbohydrates 17.0g	6%
Dietary Fiber 1.9g	8%
Sugars 6.4g	
Protein 15.8g	
Vitamin A 7%	Vitamin C 5%
Calcium 5%	Iron 7%
Nutrition Grade B-	
* Based on a 2000 calorie diet	

Ingredients
- 1 1/4 cup low-fat mayonnaise
- 1 teaspoon iodized salt
- 1 teaspoon paprika
- 1/4 teaspoon ground black pepper
- 2 1/2 cups cooked chicken meat, diced
- 1 cup sliced, seedless green grapes
- 1 cup sliced almonds
- 1/2 cup water chestnuts, chopped
- 2 tablespoons fresh parsley, chopped

- 1/4 head of iceberg lettuce, shredded

Directions

1. **Stir** together the mayonnaise, salt, paprika, and black pepper in a small bowl.
2. **Combine** the remaining ingredients in a large bowl. Add the prepared dressing and gently toss.
3. **Chill** for at least 30 minutes and serve.

2. Maple Baked Salmon

Servings: 4
Preparation time: 40 minutes
Cook time: 20 minutes
Ready in: 1 hour

Nutrition Facts

Serving Size 158 g

Amount Per Serving	
Calories 240	Calories from Fat 96
	% Daily Value*
Total Fat 10.7g	**16%**
Saturated Fat 2.2g	**11%**
Cholesterol 54mg	**18%**
Sodium 441mg	**18%**
Total Carbohydrates 15.6g	**5%**
Sugars 11.8g	
Protein 19.7g	
Vitamin A 2% •	Vitamin C 7%
Calcium 4% •	Iron 6%
Nutrition Grade B+	
* Based on a 2000 calorie diet	

Ingredients
- 1/8 teaspoon ground black pepper
- 1 pound salmon fillet
- 1/4 cup pure maple syrup
- 2 tablespoons gluten-free soy sauce (or coconut aminos)
- 1 clove garlic, minced
- 1 tablespoon fresh dill, chopped
- 1 tablespoon ginger, chopped
- 1/4 teaspoon garlic salt
- 1 pinch cayenne pepper

Directions

1. **Sprinkle** salmon with black pepper. Place salmon in a shallow glass baking dish.
2. **Combine** remaining ingredients in a small bowl.
3. **Pour** prepared marinade over salmon.
4. **Cover** and place dish in the fridge and marinate for at least 30 minutes, turning once.
5. **Preheat** oven to 400 degrees F (200 degrees C). Remove dish from the fridge and uncover.
6. **Bake** salmon for 20 minutes or until fish flakes easily with a fork. Serve warm.

3. Broiled Tilapia over Brown Rice

Servings: 8
Preparation time: 15 minutes
Cook time: 50 minutes
Ready in: 1 hour and 5 minutes

Nutrition Facts

Serving Size 289 g

Amount Per Serving

Calories 311	Calories from Fat 63
	% Daily Value*
Total Fat 7.0g	11%
Saturated Fat 2.8g	14%
Trans Fat 0.0g	
Cholesterol 44mg	15%
Sodium 385mg	16%
Total Carbohydrates 39.9g	13%
Dietary Fiber 2.1g	8%
Sugars 1.2g	
Protein 21.7g	
Vitamin A 7% •	Vitamin C 23%
Calcium 5% •	Iron 11%

Nutrition Grade B+
* Based on a 2000 calorie diet

Ingredients
- 4 cups low sodium chicken broth
- 2 cups uncooked gluten-free brown rice
- 1 small onion, chopped
- 1 small red bell pepper, chopped
- 1 teaspoon iodized salt
- 3 tablespoons low-fat mayonnaise
- 1/4 teaspoon red pepper flakes, crushed

- 1/4 teaspoon dried basil
- 1/4 teaspoon garlic powder
- 1/4 teaspoon ground black pepper
- 1/8 teaspoon onion powder
- 1/4 cup Parmesan cheese
- 1/4 cup low-fat butter, softened
- 2 tablespoons fresh lime juice
- 1 1/2 pounds tilapia fillets

Directions
1. **Pour** chicken broth into a medium saucepan put over medium-high heat, and bring to a boil.
2. **Stir** in brown rice, onion, red bell pepper, and salt. Reduce heat to low and simmer covered for 40 minutes, or until liquid is absorbed. Remove pan from heat, cover, and set aside.
3. **Preheat** the broiler. Line a broiler pan with aluminum foil.
4. **Stir** together mayonnaise, red pepper flakes, basil, garlic powder, black pepper, onion powder, Parmesan cheese, butter, and lime juice in a bowl; set aside.
5. **Place** fillets on the prepared broiler pan.
6. **Broil** tilapia fillets for 6 minutes. Remove the fillets from the oven and spoon mayonnaise mixture over the top. Broil for additional 2 minutes or until fish flakes easily with a fork.
7. **Flake** tilapia into bite-sized pieces and serve over cooked brown rice.

4. Crispy Sole Fish Fillets

Servings: 4
Serving size: 1 (5-ounce) fillet
Preparation time: 10 minutes
Cook time: 12-16 minutes
Ready in: 22 minutes

Nutrition Facts

Serving Size 215 g

Amount Per Serving

Calories 298	Calories from Fat 142
	% Daily Value*
Total Fat 15.8g	**24%**
Saturated Fat 2.1g	**10%**
Trans Fat 0.0g	
Cholesterol 113mg	**38%**
Sodium 597mg	**25%**
Total Carbohydrates 9.9g	**3%**
Sugars 1.2g	
Protein 28.1g	

| Vitamin A 2% | • | Vitamin C 1% |
| Calcium 1% | • | Iron 2% |

Nutrition Grade D+

* Based on a 2000 calorie diet

Ingredients
- 1 1/2 cups gluten-free breadcrumbs
- 1 (omega-3) egg
- 1/2 teaspoon dried onion
- 1/2 teaspoon dried parsley
- 2 tablespoons Dijon mustard
- 1/4 teaspoon ground black pepper
- 1/2 teaspoon iodized salt
- 1/4 cup extra-virgin olive oil
- 4 (5-ounce) sole fish fillets

Directions
1. **Place** breadcrumbs in a shallow dish.
2. **Combine** egg, dried onion, dried parsley, mustard, pepper, and salt in a large bowl.
3. **Heat** olive oil in a large skillet over medium-high heat.
4. **Dip** fish fillets in the egg mixture then dredge in the breadcrumbs to coat evenly.
5. **Fry** fish fillets in oil until golden brown, about 3 to 4 minutes on each side.

5. Steamed Cod and Vegetables over Brown Rice

Servings: 6
Serving size:
Preparation time: 10 minutes

Cook time: 1 hour and 10 minutes
Ready in: 1 hour and 20 minutes

Nutrition Facts

Serving Size 413 g

Amount Per Serving	
Calories 348	Calories from Fat 51
	% Daily Value*
Total Fat 5.7g	**9%**
Trans Fat 0.0g	
Cholesterol 41mg	**14%**
Sodium 695mg	**29%**
Total Carbohydrates 50.6g	**17%**
Dietary Fiber 5.0g	**20%**
Sugars 2.5g	
Protein 25.6g	
Vitamin A 131% •	Vitamin C 14%
Calcium 6% •	Iron 11%
Nutrition Grade B-	
* Based on a 2000 calorie diet	

Ingredients
- 6 (4-ounce) skinless cod fillets, sliced into 1 inch thick
- 2 cups carrots, sliced crosswise
- 1 cup green beans
- 1 cup asparagus
- 4 teaspoons fresh ginger, grated
- 2 tablespoons finely fresh flat-leaf parsley, chopped
- 4 teaspoons extra-virgin olive oil
- 1/2 teaspoon salt
- 1/8 teaspoon black pepper

Brown Rice:
- 2 cups long-grain gluten-free brown rice
- 4 cups water
- 1 teaspoon kosher salt

Directions
1. **Rinse** brown rice under cold water.
2. **Pour** water in a medium saucepan. Cover and bring to a boil over high heat. Add the rice and stir in the salt. Reduce the heat to low. Cover the saucepan and simmer for 45 to 50 minutes, or until the rice is tender. Remove pan from heat, cover and let sit to steam for 10 minutes more.

3. **Combine** carrots, green beans, and asparagus in a steamer. Place steamer in a large saucepan of boiling water. Steam vegetables covered for about 7 minutes or until tender.
4. **Transfer** vegetables to a bowl and season with 1/4 teaspoon salt. Cover to keep warm.
5. **Place** cod in the steamer and sprinkle with ginger, remaining salt, and the pepper.
6. **Steam** covered for 7 minutes or until fish is cooked through.
7. **Drizzle** olive oil over cod fillets and vegetables and sprinkle chopped parsley on top.
8. **Serve** steamed cod and veggies over cooked brown rice.

6. Creamy Gluten-free Chicken Noodle Soup

Servings: 6
Preparation time: 10 minutes
Cook time: 20 minutes
Ready in: 28 minutes

Nutrition Facts

Serving Size 492 g

Amount Per Serving

Calories 349	Calories from Fat 70
	% Daily Value*
Total Fat 7.8g	**12%**
Saturated Fat 4.1g	**20%**
Trans Fat 0.0g	
Cholesterol 42mg	**14%**
Sodium 559mg	**23%**
Total Carbohydrates 50.3g	**17%**
Dietary Fiber 4.6g	**18%**
Sugars 2.9g	
Protein 19.9g	
Vitamin A 152%	Vitamin C 37%
Calcium 9%	Iron 20%

Nutrition Grade B+
* Based on a 2000 calorie diet

Ingredients
- 6 cups low-sodium pure chicken broth
- 2 cups chicken breasts, diced
- 1/4 cup ginger, grated
- 1/2 cup mushrooms, diced
- 1 large carrot, sliced
- 1 bay leaf

- 1 bunch spinach leaves
- 1 teaspoon fresh rosemary, chopped
- 1/2 teaspoon cayenne pepper
- 3 cloves garlic, minced
- 1/4 cup fresh lemon juice
- 3 tablespoons gluten-free soy sauce
- 1/2 teaspoon freshly ground black pepper
- 1/3 cup coconut milk
- 1 cup fresh cilantro, chopped
- 10 ounce gluten-free dry flat Thai rice noodles
- 1 teaspoon raw honey, to taste

Directions
1. **Boil** the noodles in a large pot of water until al dente. Rinse with cold water, drain and set aside.
2. **Boil** chicken broth in a large pot over high heat. Add the chicken, ginger, mushrooms, carrot, and bay leaf; boil for 1 minute on High. Reduce heat to medium. Cover pot and simmer for 5-6 minutes.
3. **Stir** in spinach, rosemary, cayenne, garlic, lemon juice, soy sauce, and black pepper.
4. **Reduce** heat to low then stir in the coconut milk and honey. Place noodles in bowls then ladle the chicken soup on top. Sprinkle soup with cilantro and serve.

7. Gluten Free Chicken Piccata Pasta

Servings: 5
Preparation time: 20 minutes
Cook time: 40 minutes
Ready in: 1 hour

Nutrition Facts

Serving Size 255 g

Amount Per Serving

Calories 421 — Calories from Fat 156

	% Daily Value*
Total Fat 17.3g	**27%**
Saturated Fat 4.2g	**21%**
Trans Fat 0.0g	
Cholesterol 55mg	**18%**
Sodium 381mg	**16%**
Total Carbohydrates 36.7g	**12%**
Dietary Fiber 5.0g	**20%**
Sugars 2.2g	
Protein 27.5g	
Vitamin A 6% •	Vitamin C 13%
Calcium 5% •	Iron 15%

Nutrition Grade C-

* Based on a 2000 calorie diet

Ingredients
- 1/4 teaspoon fresh ground black pepper
- 1/3 cup almond flour
- 1/3 cup parmesan cheese, grated
- 1/4 teaspoon paprika
- 1 pound skinless, boneless chicken breast halves, pounded thin and cut into 1-inch pieces
- 1/4 cup olive oil
- 1 clove garlic, minced
- 1 1/2 cup low-sodium chicken broth
- 1/4 cup sundried tomatoes, quartered
- 1/4 cup fresh lemon juice
- 1 tablespoon thyme
- 2 tablespoons capers
- 2 tablespoons low-fat butter
- 1 (8-ounce) package gluten-free pasta
- 1/4 cup fresh basil, chopped

Directions
1. **Season** chicken with black pepper. Combine almond flour, cheese, and paprika in a shallow dish; dredge chicken pieces in flour mixture.
2. **Heat** olive oil in a large heavy skillet over medium-high heat. Add garlic and sauté until light brown. Remove garlic from skillet and set aside.

3. **Cook** the chicken pieces in olive oil for 5 minutes each side, or until brown; set aside.
4. **Boil** the chicken broth in the same skillet over high heat, about 5 minutes. Scrape pan to loosen brown bits. Stir in the sundried tomatoes, sautéed garlic, lemon juice, thyme, capers, and butter; simmer for 5 minutes.
5. **Reduce** heat to medium. Add the cooked chicken to the skillet and cook for another 15 minutes, or until the sauce thickens.
6. **Cook** pasta in a large pot of lightly salted water, uncovered for about 4 to 5 minutes, or until al dente. Drain and place onto serving plates.
7. **Pour** chicken meat sauce over pasta, and then sprinkle with chopped basil on top.

8. Tomato Fish and Veggie Stew

Servings: 6
Preparation time: 15 minutes
Cook time: 25 minutes
Ready in: 40 minutes

Nutrition Facts

Serving Size 352 g

Amount Per Serving	
Calories 245	Calories from Fat 83
	% Daily Value*
Total Fat 9.2g	14%
Saturated Fat 1.2g	6%
Trans Fat 0.0g	
Cholesterol 56mg	19%
Sodium 177mg	7%
Total Carbohydrates 19.1g	6%
Dietary Fiber 7.2g	29%
Sugars 6.6g	
Protein 24.3g	
Vitamin A 260%	Vitamin C 42%
Calcium 15%	Iron 25%

Nutrition Grade A-
* Based on a 2000 calorie diet

Ingredients
- 3 tablespoons olive oil
- 4 large cloves garlic, chopped
- 1 cup onion, chopped

- 4 cups carrots, diced
- 1 cup frozen green peas
- 1 cup tomato, diced
- 1/2 cup fresh oregano, chopped
- 1 tablespoon fennel seeds, lightly crushed
- 1 teaspoon red pepper flakes
- 2 cups low-sodium chicken broth
- 1.5 pounds cod fillets, cut into 2-inch pieces
- 1 dash iodized salt
- 1 dash pepper

Directions
1. **Place** a large pot over medium-high heat then pour olive oil into the pot. Sauté garlic and onion in olive oil for 4 minutes.
2. **Stir** in the carrots, tomato and oregano, fennel seeds, red pepper flakes, and chicken broth and simmer for 10 minutes. Stir in the green peas.
3. **Add** fish on top of the vegetables and simmer covered for another 10 minutes; season with salt and pepper.
4. **Ladle** stew into bowls and serve.

9. Cherry Chicken Lettuce Wraps

Servings: 6
Preparation time: 15 minutes
Cook time: 7-10 minutes
Ready in: 22 minutes

Nutrition Facts

Serving Size 271 g

Amount Per Serving

Calories 286	Calories from Fat 73
	% Daily Value*
Total Fat 8.1g	12%
Saturated Fat 1.2g	6%
Trans Fat 0.0g	
Cholesterol 55mg	18%
Sodium 280mg	12%
Total Carbohydrates 30.8g	10%
Dietary Fiber 2.2g	9%
Sugars 6.5g	
Protein 21.0g	
Vitamin A 97% •	Vitamin C 12%
Calcium 3% •	Iron 4%

Nutrition Grade B-

* Based on a 2000 calorie diet

Ingredients

- 2 tablespoons extra virgin olive oil, divided
- 1 1/4 pounds skinless, boneless chicken breast halves, cut into bite size pieces
- 1 tablespoon fresh ginger root, minced
- 2 tablespoons cider vinegar
- 2 tablespoons gluten-free teriyaki sauce
- 1 tablespoon raw honey
- 1 pound dark sweet cherries, pitted and halved
- 1/2 cup sundried tomatoes
- 1 1/2 cups carrots, shredded
- 1/2 cup onion, chopped
- 1/3 cup sliced walnuts, toasted
- 12 lettuce leaves

Directions
1. **Heat** 1 tablespoon olive oil in a large skillet over medium high heat.
2. **Add** ginger and chicken, sauté for about 7-10 minutes, or until cooked through. Transfer cooked chicken and ginger in a large bowl.
3. **Combine** 1 tablespoon olive oil, vinegar, teriyaki sauce and honey in a small bowl then pour into chicken mixture. Add

the rest of the ingredients, except for the lettuce, and toss gently.
4. **Spoon** mixture onto 2-ply lettuce leaves. Roll up and serve.

10. Turkey and Jasmine Rice Salad

Servings: 6
Preparation time: 20 minutes
Cook time: 15 minutes + 2 hours chill time
Ready in: 2 hours and 35 minutes

Nutrition Facts	
Serving Size 251 g	
Amount Per Serving	
Calories 432	Calories from Fat 220
	% Daily Value*
Total Fat 24.4g	38%
Saturated Fat 3.1g	15%
Trans Fat 0.0g	
Cholesterol 0mg	0%
Sodium 351mg	15%
Total Carbohydrates 34.4g	11%
Dietary Fiber 4.2g	17%
Sugars 6.9g	
Protein 20.3g	
Vitamin A 14%	Vitamin C 60%
Calcium 2%	Iron 14%
Nutrition Grade B-	
* Based on a 2000 calorie diet	

Ingredients
- 1 1/2 cups water
- 1 cup gluten-free jasmine rice
- 2 cups cooked skinless boneless turkey breast, diced
- 1 cup seedless red grapes, halved
- 3/4 pound ripe plum tomato, seeded and diced
- 1/2 cup chopped celery
- 1 cup diced green bell pepper
- 1/2 cup coarsely chopped pecans, toasted
- 1/3 cup diced red onion

Dressing:
- 1/2 cup extra virgin olive oil
- 6 tablespoons fresh cilantro, chopped
- 3 tablespoons rice vinegar
- 1 tablespoon Dijon mustard

- 1/2 teaspoon cayenne pepper
- 3/4 teaspoon iodized salt
- 3/4 teaspoon ground black pepper

Directions
1. **Place** a pot of water over medium heat and bring to a boil. Add the rice and bring to a boil again. Reduce heat to low. Cover pot and cook rice for 15 to 20 minutes, or until tender.
2. **Place** the cooked rice in a large bowl and toss in turkey, grapes, tomato, celery, bell pepper, pecans, and red onion.
3. **Combine** all the ingredients for the dressing, and toss with the salad. Cover and refrigerate salad for at least 2 hours.

11. Chicken 'N Mushroom Pasta

Servings: 7
Preparation time: 15 minutes
Cook time: 28 minutes
Ready in: 43 minutes

Nutrition Facts
Serving Size 186 g

Amount Per Serving
Calories 429 — Calories from Fat 55

	% Daily Value*
Total Fat 6.1g	9%
Saturated Fat 1.0g	5%
Trans Fat 0.0g	
Cholesterol 17mg	6%
Sodium 241mg	10%
Total Carbohydrates 73.5g	25%
Dietary Fiber 6.1g	25%
Sugars 6.6g	
Protein 13.7g	

Vitamin A 1% • Vitamin C 17%
Calcium 3% • Iron 10%

Nutrition Grade B
* Based on a 2000 calorie diet

Ingredients
- 3 cups gluten-free mostaccioli
- 2 tablespoons extra-virgin olive oil
- 3 skinless, boneless chicken breast halves
- 1 clove garlic, crushed and chopped
- 1/4 onion, chopped

- 3 fresh mushrooms, sliced
- 1 medium green bell pepper, seeded and diced
- 1/2 tablespoon dried basil
- 1/2 tablespoon dried marjoram
- 1/2 tablespoon dried oregano
- 1/2 tablespoon dried rosemary
- 2 cups ripe tomatoes, diced
- 1/2 teaspoon iodized salt
- 1/4 teaspoon pepper
- 2 tablespoons parmesan cheese, grated

Directions
1. **Cook** pasta in lightly salted water until al dente, about 8 to 10 minutes; refer to package directions for best result. Drain, cover and set aside.
2. **Heat** olive oil in a large skillet over medium heat. Add chicken and cook for 15 minutes. Remove cooked chicken from pan, let cool then dice; set aside.
3. **Sauté** garlic in the same skillet until lightly browned. Add onion, mushrooms, bell pepper, and the remaining ingredients except for the cheese; cook until mushrooms are tender.
4. **Remove** skillet from heat and add chicken and pasta; toss gently.
5. **Transfer** mixture to serving plates, sprinkle parmesan cheese on top and serve.

12. Citrus Tuna Steak Sandwich

Servings: 4
Preparation time: 10 minutes + 30 minutes marinate time
Cook time: 10 minutes
Ready in: 50 minutes

Nutrition Facts

Serving Size 332 g

Amount Per Serving

Calories 473	Calories from Fat 152
	% Daily Value*
Total Fat 16.9g	**26%**
Saturated Fat 2.4g	**12%**
Trans Fat 0.0g	
Cholesterol 32mg	**11%**
Sodium 649mg	**27%**
Total Carbohydrates 55.6g	**19%**
Dietary Fiber 2.6g	**10%**
Sugars 9.4g	
Protein 25.7g	
Vitamin A 57% •	Vitamin C 27%
Calcium 11% •	Iron 19%

Nutrition Grade B+

* Based on a 2000 calorie diet

Ingredients
- 2 tablespoons extra-virgin olive oil
- 1/4 cup gluten-free soy sauce
- 1 tablespoon lemon juice
- 1/4 cup orange juice
- 2 teaspoons raw honey
- 1/2 teaspoon dried rosemary
- 2 tablespoons fresh parsley, chopped
- 1 clove garlic, minced
- 1/4 cup green onions, chopped
- 1 dash red pepper flakes
- 1/2 teaspoon ground black pepper
- 4 (2-ounce) tuna steaks
- Olive oil for greasing
- 4 (2-ounce) gluten-free sandwich buns
- 1/4 cup gluten-free low-fat mayonnaise
- 4 lettuce leaves

Directions
1. **Place** tuna steaks in a large dish. Combine the first 11 ingredients and pour over tuna; turn to coat. Cover, and marinate in the fridge for at least 30 minutes.
2. **Grease** grill grate lightly with olive oil. Preheat grill to high heat.

3. **Cook** the tuna steaks for 5 to 6 minutes each side; baste with the marinade on each side.
4. **Spread** 1 tablespoon mayonnaise on each sandwich bun then top with the grilled tuna steak, and lettuce.

DINNER

1. Mozzarella and Spinach Stuffed Cajun Chicken

Servings: 8
Preparation time: 15 minutes
Cook time: 35-40 minutes
Ready in: 50 minutes

Nutrition Facts

Serving Size 83 g

Amount Per Serving	
Calories 191	Calories from Fat 97
	% Daily Value*
Total Fat 10.7g	17%
Saturated Fat 3.5g	18%
Cholesterol 58mg	19%
Sodium 715mg	30%
Total Carbohydrates 2.6g	1%
Dietary Fiber 0.7g	3%
Protein 20.6g	
Vitamin A 16% • Vitamin C 3%	
Calcium 13% • Iron 8%	

Nutrition Grade B-
* Based on a 2000 calorie diet

Ingredients
- 1 lb. boneless, skinless chicken breasts
- 2 teaspoon iodized salt, divided
- 2 teaspoon ground black pepper, divided
- 4 oz. mozzarella cheese, shredded
- 1 cup frozen spinach, thawed and drained
- 1 tablespoon breadcrumbs
- 2 teaspoons paprika
- 1 teaspoon garlic powder
- 1 teaspoon dried oregano

- 1 teaspoon dried thyme
- 1/2 teaspoon onion powder
- 1/2 teaspoon cayenne pepper
- 2 tablespoon extra-virgin olive oil
- Toothpicks

Directions
1. **Preheat** oven to 350 degrees F. Line a baking sheet with tin foil.
2. **Halve** chicken breasts and pound evenly to 1/4-inch thickness; season with 1 teaspoon salt and pepper.
3. **Mix** the mozzarella cheese, spinach, and remaining salt and pepper in a bowl. To make a Cajun seasoning, stir together the breadcrumbs, paprika, garlic powder, oregano, thyme, onion powder, and cayenne pepper in a separate bowl.
4. **Spoon** spinach mixture, about 1/4 cup, onto each chicken breast. Roll each chicken breast tightly and secure with toothpicks, then brush with olive oil. Sprinkle the prepared Cajun seasoning evenly over chicken breast.
5. **Place** stuffed chicken breasts onto the baking sheet. Bake for 35 to 40 minutes, or until chicken is no longer pink in the center.
6. **Slice** and serve.

2. Herbed Spaghetti Squash

Servings: 3
Preparation time: 10 minutes
Cook time: 40 minutes
Ready in: 50 minutes

Nutrition Facts

Serving Size 621 g

Amount Per Serving

Calories 358 — Calories from Fat 182

	% Daily Value*
Total Fat 20.2g	31%
Saturated Fat 7.5g	38%
Cholesterol 33mg	11%
Sodium 501mg	21%
Total Carbohydrates 41.1g	14%
Dietary Fiber 2.4g	9%
Sugars 5.0g	
Protein 9.8g	

Vitamin A 16% • Vitamin C 58%
Calcium 32% • Iron 19%

Nutrition Grade B+

* Based on a 2000 calorie diet

Ingredients
- Olive oil for greasing
- 1 (3-pound) spaghetti squash, halved lengthwise and seeded
- 2 tablespoons olive oil
- 3 cloves garlic, crushed and chopped
- 1 onion, chopped
- 1 1/2 cups tomatoes, chopped
- 2 tablespoons parsley, chopped
- 2 tablespoons sage, chopped
- 2 tablespoons chives, chopped
- 3/4 cup crumbled feta cheese

Directions
1. **Preheat** oven to 350 degrees F (175 degrees C). Lightly grease a baking sheet with olive oil.
2. **Place** spaghetti squash on the prepared baking sheet, cut sides down.
3. **Bake** for 30 minutes until tender. Remove squash from oven, let cool a bit, and set aside.
4. **Heat** olive oil in a skillet over medium heat. Add garlic and sauté until golden brown. Stir in onions and tomatoes, and cook until tomatoes are heated through.
5. **Scrape** the inside of spaghetti squash halves with a fork to a medium bowl. Add the tomato mixture, parsley, sage, chives, and feta cheese. Serve warm.

3. Turkey Veggie Stew with Toasted Bread

Servings: 4
Preparation time: 10 minutes
Cook time: 50 minutes
Ready in: 1 hour

Nutrition Facts
Serving Size 420 g

Amount Per Serving

Calories 257 Calories from Fat 49

% Daily Value*

Total Fat 5.4g	**8%**
Saturated Fat 2.2g	**11%**
Trans Fat 0.0g	
Cholesterol 33mg	**11%**
Sodium 414mg	**17%**
Total Carbohydrates 32.7g	**11%**
Dietary Fiber 5.1g	**20%**
Sugars 7.3g	
Protein 17.9g	

Vitamin A 174% • Vitamin C 79%
Calcium 9% • Iron 16%

Nutrition Grade B
* Based on a 2000 calorie diet

Ingredients
- 2 tablespoons low-fat butter
- 3 medium carrots, peeled and sliced into 1 inch pieces
- 2 medium onions, chopped
- 2 stalks celery, cut into 1 inch pieces
- 3 tablespoons gluten-free all-purpose flour
- 3 1/2 cups low-sodium chicken broth
- 1 tablespoon fresh thyme, chopped
- 1 tablespoon fresh rosemary, chopped
- 1 tablespoon fresh cilantro, minced
- 2 boneless, skinless turkey breast halves, cut into ½-inch cubes
- 1 red bell pepper, diced
- 4 large slices toasted gluten-free garlic bread

Directions
1. **Place** a pot over medium heat. Add butter and melt. Add carrots, onions, celery and sauté until tender. Stir in the

chicken broth and flour, season with thyme, rosemary, and cilantro.
2. **Add** turkey and bring to a boil.
3. **Reduce** heat to low, and simmer covered for 30 minutes.
4. **Add** green bell pepper and cook 10 minutes more, until pepper is tender.
5. **Serve** warm with toasted garlic bread.

4. Grilled Sea Bass with Lemon Fettuccine

Servings: 8
Preparation time: 15 minutes
Cook time: 26 minutes
Ready in: 41 minutes

Nutrition Facts

Serving Size 238 g

Amount Per Serving	
Calories 291	Calories from Fat 62
	% Daily Value*
Total Fat 6.9g	**11%**
Saturated Fat 1.4g	7%
Trans Fat 0.0g	
Cholesterol 84mg	**28%**
Sodium 1245mg	**52%**
Total Carbohydrates 37.3g	**12%**
Dietary Fiber 4.0g	**16%**
Sugars 4.3g	
Protein 20.5g	
Vitamin A 8%	Vitamin C 18%
Calcium 6%	Iron 6%

Nutrition Grade C-
* Based on a 2000 calorie diet

Ingredients
- 1/2 cup fresh parsley, chopped
- 1/4 cup parmesan cheese, grated
- 2 tablespoon lemon zest
- 1/4 cup fresh lemon juice
- 16 ounce gluten-free fettuccine
- 1/2 teaspoon iodized salt
- 1/4 teaspoon ground black pepper
- 1/4 teaspoon onion powder
- 1/4 teaspoon paprika
- 1/4 teaspoon garlic powder

- 1/4 teaspoon cayenne pepper
- 1/2 teaspoon iodized salt
- 1 lemon, juiced
- 2 pounds sea bass fillets
- 5 tablespoons extra virgin olive oil
- 2 large cloves garlic, chopped
- 1 tablespoon cilantro, chopped

Directions
1. **Stir** together the parsley, cheese, lemon zest, and lemon juice in a large bowl.
2. **Cook** fettuccine until al dente; refer to package directions. Drain and toss with the lemon mixture in the large bowl. Season with salt and black pepper. Set aside.
3. **Preheat** grill to high heat.
4. **Mix** the onion powder, paprika, garlic powder, cayenne pepper, and salt. Rub seasonings onto the fish and drizzle with lemon juice and 1 tablespoon olive oil.
5. **Heat** 2 tablespoons olive oil in a saucepan over medium heat. Add the garlic and cilantro, sauté until garlic is lightly browned; set aside.
6. **Grease** grill grate lightly with 1 tablespoon olive oil. Grill fish for 7 minutes each side, or until fish flakes easily with a fork.
7. **Divide** cooked lemon fettuccine among serving plates and top with the fillets. Top fillets with sautéed garlic and cilantro then drizzle with remaining olive oil before serving.

5. Gluten-free Chicken and Veggie Stir Fry

Servings: 8
Preparation time: 15 minutes
Cook time: 20 minutes
Ready in: 35 minutes

Nutrition Facts

Serving Size 175 g

Amount Per Serving

Calories 220   Calories from Fat 106

% Daily Value*

Total Fat 11.8g	**18%**
Saturated Fat 2.5g	**12%**
Trans Fat 0.0g	
Cholesterol 50mg	**17%**
Sodium 363mg	**15%**
Total Carbohydrates 9.5g	**3%**
Dietary Fiber 1.9g	**7%**
Sugars 3.2g	
Protein 19.2g	

Vitamin A 96% • Vitamin C 12%
Calcium 3% • Iron 8%

Nutrition Grade B

* Based on a 2000 calorie diet

Ingredients
- 1 pound boneless chicken breast cut into 1 inch pieces
- 2 tablespoons extra-virgin olive oil
- 2 cups carrots, sliced
- 1 onion, chopped
- 2 cloves garlic, minced
- 1/2 cup snap peas
- 1/2 cup low-sodium pure chicken broth
- 3 tablespoon gluten-free organic soy sauce
- 1/4 teaspoon ground black pepper, or to taste
- ½ teaspoon raw honey
- 1/4 teaspoon red pepper flakes
- 1 thumbs-size ginger, grated
- 1 teaspoon arrowroot powder dissolved in 1 teaspoon water
- 1/2 cup fresh cilantro, chopped
- 1/2 cup cashews, chopped

Directions
1. **Heat** olive oil in a medium saucepan over medium heat. Add the garlic and sauté until lightly brown.
2. **Add** the chicken and onions, cook for 5 minutes.
3. **Stir** in the carrots and snap peas and cook for an additional 8 minutes. Add chicken broth, soy sauce, honey, ginger, red pepper flakes, and black pepper. Simmer covered for 5

minutes. Stir in dissolved arrowroot powder and simmer until sauce thickens.
4. **Place** dish in individual plates and serve topped with chopped cilantro and cashews.

6. Grilled Spicy Cod with Honey Roasted Carrots

Servings: 4
Preparation time: 15 minutes
Cook time: 1 hour and 10 minutes
Ready in: 1 hour and 25 minutes

Nutrition Facts
Serving Size 311 g

Amount Per Serving	
Calories 369	Calories from Fat 75
	% Daily Value*
Total Fat 8.3g	**13%**
Saturated Fat 1.0g	**5%**
Trans Fat 0.0g	
Cholesterol 56mg	**19%**
Sodium 1158mg	**48%**
Total Carbohydrates 37.0g	**12%**
Dietary Fiber 5.3g	**21%**
Sugars 27.5g	
Protein 21.8g	
Vitamin A 311%	Vitamin C 12%
Calcium 8%	Iron 12%
Nutrition Grade B-	
* Based on a 2000 calorie diet	

Ingredients
- 6 carrots, peeled
- 2 tablespoons extra-virgin olive oil
- 1/3 cup raw honey
- 1/2 teaspoon iodized salt
- 1/4 teaspoon ground black pepper
- Olive oil for greasing
- 1 pounds cod fillets, rinsed and patted dry
- 1 1/2 cups organic low-sodium chunky salsa
- 2 tablespoons fresh cilantro, chopped
- 1/2 cup olive tapenade
- 1/2 teaspoon iodized salt
- 1/2 teaspoon pepper to taste

Directions
1. **Preheat** oven to 350 degrees F (175 degrees C).
2. **Place** the whole carrots into a baking dish, and drizzle with olive oil; turn to coat. Pour the honey over carrots, then sprinkle with salt and pepper; mix until evenly coated.
3. **Bake** for 40 minutes, or until just tender. Remove from oven, cover and set aside.
4. **Lightly** grease a baking dish with olive oil. Place fillets in the baking dish.
5. **Season** fillets with salt and pepper.
6. **Pour** salsa and olive tapenade over fish and sprinkle with chopped cilantro.
7. **Bake** for 30 minutes. Place fish onto individual plates then add the honey roasted carrots on the side.

7. Pork Chops in Raspberry Sauce with Herbed Basmati Rice

Servings: 4

Serving size: 1 (4-ounce) pork chop and 1 cup herbed basmati rice

Preparation time: 15 minutes

Cook time: 26 minutes

Ready in: 41 minutes

Nutrition Facts

Serving Size 323 g

Amount Per Serving	
Calories 447	Calories from Fat 134
	% Daily Value*
Total Fat 14.8g	23%
Saturated Fat 5.2g	26%
Trans Fat 0.0g	
Cholesterol 61mg	20%
Sodium 1125mg	47%
Total Carbohydrates 51.7g	17%
Dietary Fiber 1.7g	7%
Sugars 12.8g	
Protein 24.9g	
Vitamin A 6%	Vitamin C 19%
Calcium 5%	Iron 10%
Nutrition Grade D+	
* Based on a 2000 calorie diet	

Ingredients

Herbed Basmati Rice:
- 1 cup uncooked long-grain gluten-free white basmati rice
- 1 3/4 cups water
- 3/4 teaspoon iodized salt
- 1 tablespoon unsalted butter
- 1 garlic clove, crushed and chopped
- 2 tablespoons fresh parsley leaves, minced
- 3 tablespoons fresh green onions, chopped
- 1 shallot, minced
- 1/4 teaspoon freshly ground black pepper

Pork Chops:
- 1/2 teaspoon dried rosemary, crushed
- 1/2 teaspoon dried thyme, crushed
- 1/2 teaspoon dried sage, crushed
- 1/4 teaspoon iodized salt
- 1/4 teaspoon ground black pepper
- 4 (4 ounce) lean boneless pork loin chops
- 1 tablespoon low-fat butter
- 1 tablespoon extra-virgin olive oil
- 1/4 cup seedless raspberry jam
- 2 tablespoons freshly squeezed lemon juice
- 1 teaspoon raw honey
- 2 tablespoons balsamic vinegar

Directions
1. **Heat** water in a small saucepan over high heat. Add the rice, salt, and butter, and bring to a boil.
2. **Turn** heat to low and stir once. Cover saucepan and simmer for 15 minutes. Remove from heat and let sit for 5 minutes.
3. **Stir** in the garlic, parsley, green onions, shallot, and pepper; fluff with a fork, cover and set aside.
4. **Mix** rosemary, thyme, sage, salt, and pepper, and then rub evenly over pork chops.
5. **Place** a nonstick skillet over medium-high heat. Add the butter and olive oil. Once the butter is melted, add the pork chops and cook for 4 to 5 minutes on each side.
6. **Remove** pork chops to a plate and cover to keep warm.
7. **Stir** together raspberry jam, lemon juice, honey, and vinegar in the skillet and bring to a boil. Simmer sauce for 2 to 3 minutes, or until it starts to thicken.

8. **Spoon** sauce in a pool onto a serving plate, and top with pork chops. Serve with herbed basmati rice.

8. Teriyaki Salmon with Jasmine Rice

Servings: 6
Preparation time: 10 minutes
Cook time: 25 minutes + 30 minutes marinate time
Ready in: 1 hour and 5 minutes

Nutrition Facts

Serving Size 302 g

Amount Per Serving

Calories 405	Calories from Fat 93
	% Daily Value*
Total Fat 10.4g	**16%**
Saturated Fat 2.2g	**11%**
Cholesterol 48mg	**16%**
Sodium 798mg	**33%**
Total Carbohydrates 54.0g	**18%**
Dietary Fiber 3.2g	**13%**
Sugars 3.7g	
Protein 21.8g	
Vitamin A 3%	Vitamin C 24%
Calcium 3%	Iron 15%

Nutrition Grade B
* Based on a 2000 calorie diet

Ingredients
- 2 cups gluten-free jasmine rice
- 3 cups water
- 1 teaspoon iodized salt
- 1 pound salmon
- 1/4 cup gluten-free low-sodium soy sauce
- 1 teaspoon extra-virgin olive oil
- 1/2 cup lemon juice
- 1 tablespoon raw honey
- 1 teaspoon ground mustard
- 1 tablespoon ginger, minced
- 2 cloves garlic, minced
- 1/2 cup scallions, finely chopped
- 1/4 teaspoon ground black pepper
- 1 lemongrass leaf, minced

Directions
1. **Rinse** rice with cold water.
2. **Heat** water in a saucepan. Add rice and salt then bring to a boil. Reduce heat to low and cover pan.
3. **Cook** rice for 10 to 12 minutes, or until tender. Remove from heat and let stand for 5 minutes; fluff with a fork.
4. **Preheat** the oven to 350 degrees F. Line a baking sheet with grease-proof paper.
5. **Place** salmon in a large dish. Stir together the remaining ingredients and pour over salmon.
6. **Marinate** in the fridge for at least 30 minutes. Transfer salmon to the baking sheet.
7. **Bake** for 10-12 minutes, or until just cooked. Serve with jasmine rice.

9. Gluten-Free Turkey Meat Loaf

Servings: 6
Preparation time: 15 minutes
Cook time: 1hour and 30 minutes
Ready in: 1hour and 45 minutes

Nutrition Facts
Serving Size 166 g

Amount Per Serving	
Calories 251	Calories from Fat 107
	% Daily Value*
Total Fat 11.9g	18%
Saturated Fat 3.3g	16%
Trans Fat 0.0g	
Cholesterol 125mg	42%
Sodium 480mg	20%
Total Carbohydrates 12.7g	4%
Dietary Fiber 5.0g	20%
Sugars 5.0g	
Protein 22.3g	
Vitamin A 13%	Vitamin C 17%
Calcium 7%	Iron 17%
Nutrition Grade B-	
* Based on a 2000 calorie diet	

Ingredients
- 1 tablespoon olive oil
- 1 onion, diced
- 1 1/4 pound lean ground turkey

- 2 (omega-3) eggs, beaten
- 1/2 cup coconut flour
- 1/4 cup fresh thyme, chopped
- 2 tablespoons dried rosemary
- 1/2 cup fresh parsley, chopped
- 1 teaspoon ground coriander
- 1/2 teaspoon iodized salt
- 1/2 teaspoon ground black pepper
- 1/3 cup gluten-free ketchup

Directions
1. **Preheat** oven to 350° F. Prepare a parchment-lined 9 x 5-inch loaf pan.
2. **Heat** olive oil in a small skillet or pan over medium-low heat. Add the onion and sauté until soft. Remove from heat and set aside.
3. **Place** turkey in a large bowl. Add the sautéed onion, eggs, coconut flour, thyme, rosemary, parsley, cumin, salt, and pepper. Place mixture in the loaf pan and spread ketchup evenly over the top.
4. **Bake** for 1 hour and 30 minutes, or until internal temperature reaches 160 degrees F. Let cool, slice and serve with ketchup.

10. Zesty Olive Chicken with Fried Rice

Servings: 4
Preparation time: 15 minutes
Cook time: 45 minutes
Ready in: 1 hour

Nutrition Facts

Serving Size 305 g

Amount Per Serving

Calories 411	Calories from Fat 178
	% Daily Value*
Total Fat 19.8g	**30%**
Saturated Fat 3.0g	**15%**
Cholesterol 33mg	**11%**
Sodium 770mg	**32%**
Total Carbohydrates 41.2g	**14%**
Dietary Fiber 1.6g	**6%**
Sugars 1.0g	
Protein 16.6g	
Vitamin A 13% •	Vitamin C 14%
Calcium 4% •	Iron 15%

Nutrition Grade C+

* Based on a 2000 calorie diet

Ingredients
- 1 cup gluten-free white rice
- 2 cups water
- 1/3 cup baby carrots, chopped
- 1/4 cup frozen green peas
- 1 tablespoon extra-virgin olive oil
- 1 tablespoon gluten-free, low-sodium soy sauce
- 4 skinless, boneless chicken breast halves (about 2 (4-ounce) chicken breast fillets)
- 1/2 teaspoon iodized salt
- 1/2 teaspoon ground black pepper
- 4 tablespoons extra-virgin olive oil
- 3 cloves garlic, chopped
- 1 medium shallot, chopped
- 1 cup low-sodium pure chicken broth
- 2 tablespoons lemon juice
- 1/4 cup green olives, halved

Directions
1. **Boil** rice and water in a saucepan over medium heat. Reduce heat to low. Simmer covered for 20 minutes.
2. **Boil** carrots and peas in water for 3 to 5 minutes. Drain well.
3. **Heat** olive oil in a wok over high heat. Add the carrots, peas, and cooked rice; drizzle with soy sauce, and toss to coat. Cook for about 5 minutes, remove from heat and set aside.

4. **Season** chicken with salt and pepper.
5. **Place** a large skillet over medium-high heat then pour in 2 tablespoons olive oil. Once oil is hot, add the chicken and cook for 5 minutes on each side, or until golden brown.
6. **Reduce** heat to medium, and pour the remaining olive oil in the same skillet.
7. **Sauté** garlic and shallot in olive oil until garlic is lightly browned. Stir in chicken broth, lemon juice, and olives. Simmer for 5 to 10 minutes, or until the sauce thickens and juice is absorbed.
8. **Serve** with fried rice.

11. Ultimate Spicy Orange Chicken

Servings: 4
Serving size: 1 chicken breast half and 1/2 cup cooked rice
Preparation time: 10 minutes
Cook time: 15 minutes
Ready in: 25 minutes

Nutrition Facts

Serving Size 271 g

Amount Per Serving	
Calories 572	Calories from Fat 136
	% Daily Value*
Total Fat 15.1g	23%
Saturated Fat 2.4g	12%
Trans Fat 0.0g	
Cholesterol 49mg	16%
Sodium 289mg	12%
Total Carbohydrates 82.1g	27%
Dietary Fiber 4.0g	16%
Sugars 5.7g	
Protein 25.3g	
Vitamin A 4%	Vitamin C 65%
Calcium 5%	Iron 12%

Nutrition Grade B+
* Based on a 2000 calorie diet

Ingredients
- 1/8 teaspoon ground thyme
- 1/4 teaspoon onion powder
- 1/4 teaspoon garlic powder
- 1/4 teaspoon iodized salt
- 1/4 teaspoon ground black pepper

- 3 tablespoons extra-virgin olive oil
- 4 (3-ounce) skinless, boneless chicken breast halves
- 1 cup orange juice
- 1 lemon, juiced
- 1/4 teaspoon red pepper flakes
- 1/4 teaspoon ground cinnamon
- 1 teaspoon fresh basil, chopped
- 1/2 teaspoon ground ginger
- 2 teaspoons cornstarch, dissolved in 1 tablespoon water
- 2 cups cooked gluten-free brown rice

Directions
1. **Combine** thyme, onion powder, garlic powder, salt, and pepper in a small bowl then rub into chicken breast halves.
2. **Heat** the olive oil in a medium skillet over medium heat. Cook chicken 5 to 10 minutes on each side, or until no longer pink inside. Transfer to a large dish and set aside.
3. **Stir** together the orange juice, lemon juice, red pepper flakes, cinnamon, basil, ginger, and cornstarch mixture in the same skillet over high heat.
4. **Cook** for 4 to 5 minutes, until thickened; stirring continuously. Spoon sauce over cooked chicken breast halves.
5. **Serve** warm with brown rice.

12. Creamy Chicken and Wild Rice Soup

Servings: 5
Preparation time: 10 minutes
Cook time: 41 minutes
Ready in: 25

Nutrition Facts

Serving Size 525 g

Amount Per Serving

Calories 390   Calories from Fat 125

                                                    % Daily Value*

	% Daily Value*
Total Fat 13.8g	**21%**
Saturated Fat 4.9g	**25%**
Trans Fat 0.0g	
Cholesterol 21mg	**7%**
Sodium 809mg	**34%**
Total Carbohydrates 47.6g	**16%**
Dietary Fiber 3.8g	**15%**
Sugars 6.8g	
Protein 19.1g	

Vitamin A 42% • Vitamin C 5%
Calcium 13% • Iron 4%

Nutrition Grade C+

* Based on a 2000 calorie diet

Ingredients

- 1 tablespoon extra-virgin olive oil
- 3 cloves garlic, crushed and chopped
- 1/2 cup onion, minced
- 1/2 cup carrots, diced
- 1/2 cup celery, diced
- 4 cups low-sodium chicken broth
- 2 cups water
- 1 (8-ounce) cooked, chicken breast fillet, shredded
- 1 (4.5 ounce) package quick cooking gluten-free long grain and wild rice
- 1/2 teaspoon iodized salt
- 1/2 teaspoon ground black pepper
- 1/2 cup gluten-free all-purpose flour
- 6 tablespoons low-fat butter
- 2 cups 1% milk

Directions

1. **Heat** olive oil in a large saucepan over medium heat. Add garlic and sauté until golden brown. Stir in the onions and cook until soft. Add the carrots and celery and cook for about 6 minutes, or until softened.
2. **Pour** in chicken broth, water and chicken. Bring to a boil then stir in wild rice. Reduce heat to medium-low. Cover and

simmer for 20 minutes, or until rice is tender and slightly firm. Remove from heat and set aside.
3. **Mix** salt, pepper, and flour in a small bowl. Melt butter in a medium saucepan over medium heat. Reduce heat to low, and then add the flour mixture. Gradually add milk; stirring continuously until smooth. Simmer for 5 minutes until soup is thick.
4. **Pour** milk mixture over cooked chicken and rice mixture. Simmer for 10 to 15 minutes over medium heat. Serve warm.

DESSERT

1. Peach and Triple Berry Parfaits

Servings: 6
Preparation time: 15 minutes

Nutrition Facts
Serving Size 235 g

Amount Per Serving
Calories 319   Calories from Fat 179
                           % Daily Value*
Total Fat 19.9g   31%
  Saturated Fat 1.8g   9%
Cholesterol 1mg   0%
Sodium 30mg   1%
Total Carbohydrates 30.6g   10%
  Dietary Fiber 6.5g   26%
  Sugars 19.7g
Protein 9.8g

Vitamin A 15%   •   Vitamin C 88%
Calcium 6%   •   Iron 9%

Nutrition Grade A-
* Based on a 2000 calorie diet

Ingredients
- 2 peaches, peeled, pitted, and sliced into 2 1/2-inch pieces
- 1 1/2 cups fresh strawberries, stemmed and sliced
- 1 cup fresh blueberries
- 1 cup fresh raspberries
- 1 tablespoon raw honey
- 1 tablespoon lemon juice
- 2 cups reduced-fat organic coconut cream
- 1 cup walnuts, sliced

Directions
1. **Chill** a mixing bowl and 4 parfait glasses.
2. **Place** coconut cream into a pre-chilled mixing bowl and beat on High using a handheld blender until thick and peaks form.
3. **Combine** the peaches and berries in a bowl; drizzle with honey and lemon juice, gently toss to coat.
4. **Layer** the fruits with coconut cream and walnuts in the parfait glasses. Chill and serve.

2. Mixed Triple Berry Crisp

Servings: 6
Preparation time: 10 minutes
Cook time: 30-35 minutes
Ready in: 1 hour

Nutrition Facts
Serving Size 187 g

Amount Per Serving
Calories 425   Calories from Fat 205
                              % Daily Value*
Total Fat 22.8g   35%
  Saturated Fat 7.8g   39%
  Trans Fat 0.0g
Cholesterol 0mg   0%
Sodium 152mg   6%
Total Carbohydrates 50.1g   17%
  Dietary Fiber 9.6g   39%
  Sugars 19.7g
Protein 10.4g

Vitamin A 2%   •   Vitamin C 27%
Calcium 3%   •   Iron 17%
Nutrition Grade C-
* Based on a 2000 calorie diet

Ingredients
- 1 cup chopped walnuts
- 1 1/2 cups gluten-free all-purpose flour
- 1 cup shredded unsweetened coconut
- 1 teaspoon cinnamon
- 1/4 teaspoon iodized salt
- 1/4 cup raw honey
- 1 teaspoon pure vanilla extract
- 1/3 cup low-fat butter, melted
- 2 cups fresh blueberries

- 1 cup fresh blackberries
- 1 cup fresh raspberries

Directions
1. **Preheat** oven to 350 degrees F (175 degrees C). Grease an 8x8 inch baking pan with coconut oil.
2. **Make** the topping: combine walnuts, flour, shredded coconut, cinnamon, and salt in a large bowl. Drizzle the mixture with honey and vanilla, add butter then toss to coat.
3. **Mix** all the berries then place in the baking pan. Spoon the prepared crumble topping over the top.
4. **Bake** for about 30-35 minutes.

3. Pumpkin Protein Cookies

Servings: 4
Serving size: 3 cookies
Preparation time: 15 minutes
Cook time: 5-10 minutes
Ready in: 20 minutes

Nutrition Facts

Serving Size 174 g

Amount Per Serving	
Calories 418	Calories from Fat 154
	% Daily Value*
Total Fat 17.1g	26%
Saturated Fat 1.6g	8%
Trans Fat 0.0g	
Cholesterol 0mg	0%
Sodium 858mg	36%
Total Carbohydrates 56.9g	19%
Dietary Fiber 10.9g	44%
Sugars 20.2g	
Protein 12.0g	
Vitamin A 191% •	Vitamin C 5%
Calcium 8% •	Iron 13%
Nutrition Grade B	
* Based on a 2000 calorie diet	

Ingredients
- 1/4 cup raw honey
- 1 cup gluten-free rolled oats
- 1 cup almond flour
- 1/2 cup gluten-free millet flour

- 1 3/4 teaspoons baking soda
- 1/2 teaspoon baking powder
- 1/2 teaspoon iodized salt
- 2 teaspoons ground cinnamon
- 1 teaspoon ground nutmeg
- 1 cup pumpkin puree
- 1 tablespoon applesauce
- 2 tablespoons ground flax seed mixed with 6 tablespoons water
- 1/2 teaspoon allspice

Directions
1. **Preheat** oven to 350 degrees F (175 degrees C).
2. **Gradually** combine all the ingredients in a large bowl. Divide batter into 12 balls and flatten on a baking sheet; placing 2 inches apart.
3. **Bake** for 5 minutes.

4. Cranberry Peach Pie

Servings: 8
Preparation time: 10 minutes
Cook time: 45 minutes
Ready in: 55 minutes

Nutrition Facts

Serving Size 178 g

Amount Per Serving	
Calories 342	Calories from Fat 139
	% Daily Value*
Total Fat 15.4g	24%
Saturated Fat 6.9g	35%
Trans Fat 0.0g	
Cholesterol 9mg	3%
Sodium 281mg	12%
Total Carbohydrates 52.4g	17%
Dietary Fiber 2.4g	10%
Sugars 25.2g	
Protein 3.5g	
Vitamin A 6% •	Vitamin C 12%
Calcium 1% •	Iron 2%

Nutrition Grade F
* Based on a 2000 calorie diet

Ingredients

- 4 cups fresh peaches - peeled, pitted, and sliced
- 1 cup fresh cranberries
- 1 cup chopped pecans
- 3 tablespoons gluten-free all-purpose flour
- 1/2 cup raw honey
- 1 teaspoon ground cinnamon
- 1 teaspoon pure vanilla extract
- 9-inch gluten-free double-crusts pie (recommended: Pillsbury)
- 2 tablespoons low-fat butter, softened and cut into pieces

Directions

1. **Preheat** oven to 400 degrees F (200 degrees C).
2. **Place** fruits and pecans in a large bowl.
3. **Combine** flour, honey, cinnamon, and vanilla then toss together with the fruit mixture.
4. **Line** a 9-inch pie plate with bottom pie crust. Add fruit mixture and dot with butter. Roll out remaining crust on top. Seal edges.
5. **Bake** for 45 minutes, until crust is golden brown.

Books by Maggie Fitzgerald

[The 14 Day Green Smoothie Detox Diet](#)

[The New Green Smoothie Diet](#)

[The 3-Step Thyroid Plan](#)

[www.amazon.com/author/maggiefitzgerald](#)

About Maggie Fitzgerald

Maggie Fitzgerald is a natural health, diet and nutrition expert and author from California. She has dedicated a large part of the last two decades studying and researching the amazing health benefits of green and raw diets.

She has three children and a loving husband. In her spare time she is an avid cook and enjoys hosting monthly dinner parties for her friends and family.

Exclusive Bonus Download: The Absolute Truth About Detoxification And Weight Loss!

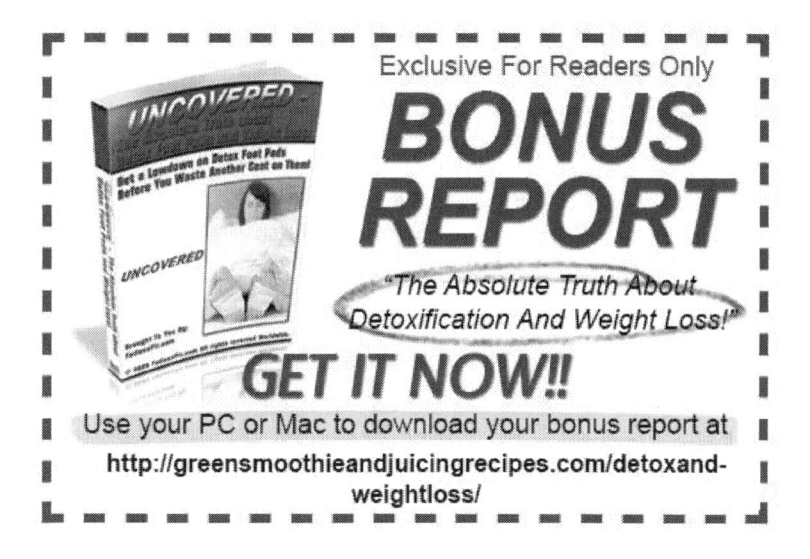

```
┌────────────────────────────────────────────┐
│              Exclusive For Readers Only    │
│   UNCOVERED                                │
│                  BONUS                     │
│                  REPORT                    │
│              "The Absolute Truth About     │
│              Detoxification And Weight Loss!"│
│              GET IT NOW!!                  │
│  Use your PC or Mac to download your bonus report at │
│   http://greensmoothieandjuicingrecipes.com/detoxand-│
│                  weightloss/               │
└────────────────────────────────────────────┘
```

Download your bonus, please visit the download link above from your PC or MAC. To open PDF files, visit http://get.adobe.com/reader/ to download the reader if it's not already installed on your PC or Mac. To open ZIP files, you may need to download WinZip from http://www.winzip.com. This download is for PC or Mac ONLY and might not be downloadable to kindle.

Detoxifying the body is very important for its health and general well-being; yet, the concept is gravely misunderstood by most people. Centuries ago, health masters in the East understood the importance of balancing and detoxifying the body. In contrast, the concept is fairly new to the practitioners of Western medicine!

As the concept of detoxification is becoming popular amount the masses, so are the myths and misinformation concerning its benefits and procedure! Unscrupulous, money-hungry manufacturers of health products aren't making the issue any less confusing for the public.

If you've heard of detoxification and are confused about the conflicting messages out there, this report is the right guide for you!

In this Report, You will discover:

- Why is Detoxification Important?!

- How Detoxification Leads to Weight Loss!

- Do Detox Diets Work?

- Do Detox Foot Pads Work?

- Do You Really Need Detox Diets and Foot Patches?

- Free and Natural Ways to Detoxify Your Body.

And MUCH MUCH MORE!

Visit the URL above to download this guide and start shredding fat NOW

One Last Thing...

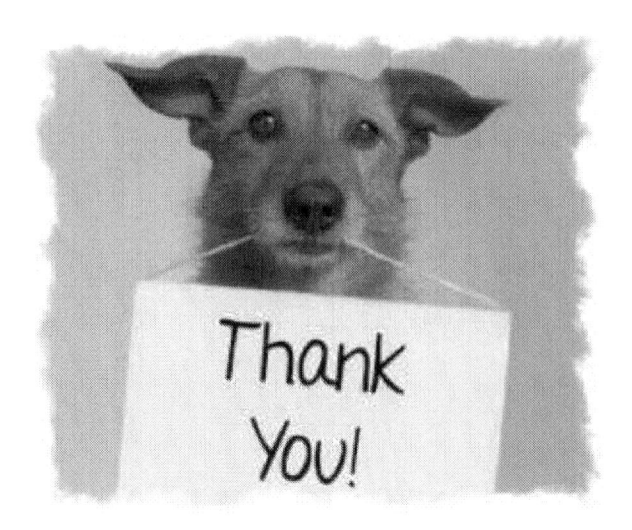

Thank you so much for reading my book. I hope you really liked it. As you probably know, many people look at the reviews on Amazon before they decide to purchase a book. If you liked the book, could you please take a minute to leave a review with your feedback? 60 seconds is all I'm asking for, and it would mean the world to me.

Maggie Fitzgerald

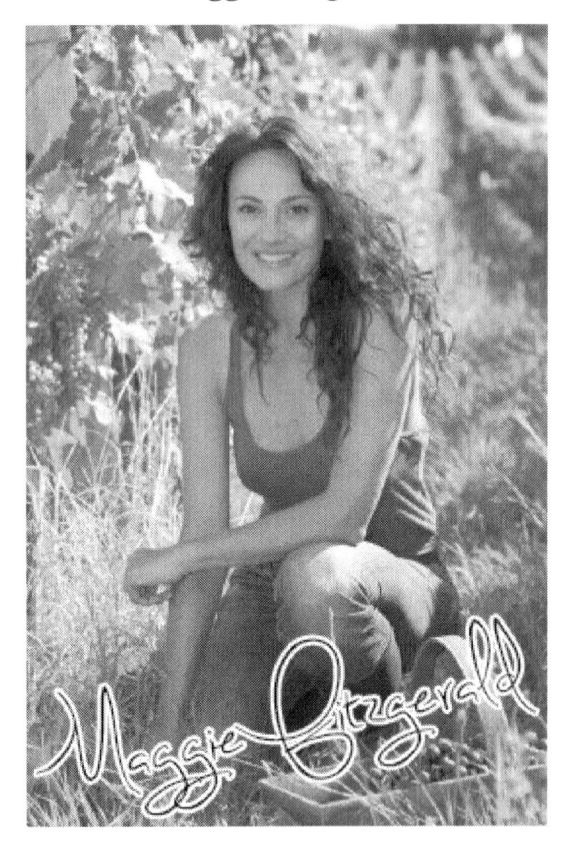

Copyright © 2012 Maggie Fitzgerald

Images and Cover by Live Natural Press

LiveNatural
PRESS

Atlanta, Georgia USA